Better partnership working

WORKING IN TEAMS

Better partnership working

Series editors: Jon Glasby and Helen Dickinson

About the authors

Kim Jelphs works as an organisational development (OD) and leadership consultant in an NHS Foundation Trust and with a wide range of organisations across sectors and agencies. She holds Honorary and Associate roles with a range of universities in the UK and Australia. Her wide-ranging consultancy experience, together with 30 years of working in the NHS holding senior clinical and managerial posts in mental health, the acute and primary care sectors, has fashioned her enthusiasm and learning in working with and developing effective team and interteam working.

Helen Dickinson is Associate Professor of Public Governance at the School of Social and Political Sciences and Melbourne School of Government, University of Melbourne, Australia. Her expertise is in public services, particularly in relation to topics such as governance, commissioning and priority setting and decision-making, and she has published widely on these topics. Helen is co-editor of the *Journal of Health, Organization and Management* and the *Australian Journal of Public Administration*. Helen has worked with a range of different levels of government, community organisations and private organisations in Australia, the UK, New Zealand and Europe on research and consultancy programmes.

Robin Miller is Senior Fellow and Director of Evaluation at the Health Services Management Centre (HSMC), Birmingham, and a Fellow of the School for Social Care Research, London, UK. He leads on a variety of applied research projects with health and social care organisations, with a particular focus on evaluating and learning from change initiatives. Robin is co-editor of the *Journal of Integrated Care* and an advisory group member of the European Primary Care Network. Prior to his academic career Robin spent 20 years as a social worker, manager and commissioner of health and social care services.

WORKING IN TEAMS

Kim Jelphs, Helen Dickinson and Robin Miller

Second Edition

First edition published in 2008

This edition published in Great Britain in 2016 by

Policy Press
University of Bristol
1-9 Old Park Hill
Bristol BS8 1SD
UK
t: +44 (0)117 954 5940
pp-info@bristol.ac.uk
www.policypress.co.uk

North America office:
Policy Press
c/o The University of Chicago Press
1427 East 60th Street
Chicago, IL 60637, USA
t: +1 773 702 7700
f: +1 773 702 9756
sales@press.uchicago.edu
www.press.uchicago.edu

© Policy Press 2016

British Library Cataloguing in Publication Data
A catalogue record for this book is available from the British Library

Library of Congress Cataloging-in-Publication Data
A catalog record for this book has been requested

ISBN 978-1-4473-2988-6 paperback
ISBN 978-1-4473-2991-6 ePub
ISBN 978-1-4473-2990-9 Mobi

The right of Kim Jelphs, Helen Dickinson and Robin Miller to be identified
as authors of this work has been asserted by them in accordance with the 1988
Copyright, Designs and Patents Act.

Cover design by Policy Press
Printed and bound in Great Britain by Lavenham Press Ltd, Suffolk
Policy Press use environmentally responsible print partners

Contents

List of tables, figures and boxes

Tables

Figures

Boxes

Acknowledgements

Kim, Helen and Robin would like to acknowledge the contribution of a number of people who allowed them to draw on and use their work in this book. Special thanks go to the following people/organisations, and also to everyone who allowed them to reproduce their stories and ideas:

- Jennie Collier, from South Staffordshire and Shropshire Healthcare NHS Foundation Trust, who provided the example in Box 1.6.
- Sunderland Clinical Commissioning Group, for the example/case study in Box 3.1.
- The Royal College of Psychiatrists, for permission to use text from Haigh (2004) on pages 50 and 51.
- Figure 3.1, from Kilmann and Thomas (1977), was reproduced with permission from the publisher, CPP, Inc. Copyright 1977. All rights reserved. Further reproduction is prohibited without CPP's written consent. For more information, please visit www.cpp.com
- Table 3.1 was based on work from Reason (2013).
- Steve Becsi (Pulse Australasia) and S. McDonald provided the example in Box 3.4.
- Table 4.1 was reproduced by kind permission of Belbin® (www.belbin.com).
- Figure 4.1 was reproduced by kind permission of Richard Boston (www.leader-space.com).
- Table 4.2, Figures 4.6 and 4.7 and Box 4.4, as well as advice on the text, were kindly provided by Lynn Markiewicz, at Aston OD.
- All efforts were made to secure permission for the use of Figure 4.2 from Edward de Bono.
- Box 4.2 and Figure 4.3 were reproduced by kind permission of Michael Leonard.
- Nancy Kline allowed the authors to use the Thinking Environment® meeting as an example, and provided advice on the text in Chapter 4 as well as the text in Box 4.3.

- Figure 4.4 was reproduced with permission from Patrick Lencioni and The Table Group.
- Figure 4.5 was reproduced from Johnson, Gerry, Scholes, Kevan and Whittington, Richard, *Exploring corporate strategy: Text and cases* (8th edn), © 2008, pp 198, 199, by permission of Pearson Education, Inc, New York.
- Table 4.3 was reproduced with thanks to M. Minkman et al (2009).

The authors' thanks also go to George Cox for his assistance in the final stages of the book in terms of formatting and bringing together the references, and to all those who read and commented on previous drafts.

Any personal opinions (or errors) in the book are those of the authors.

List of abbreviations

Health and social care use a large number of abbreviations and acronyms, and we note that a number of teams are starting to recognise that their use may potentially damage or obstruct communication. So in this text we recommend that wherever possible, abbreviations should not be used, or that when used, this is on the basis that all individuals understand these and interpret them in the same way. Inevitably, however, we have had to incorporate some abbreviations, and the more popular terms used are set out below:

BMA	British Medical Association
BMJ	*British Medical Journal*
CAHMS	Child and Adolescent Mental Health Services
CIPD	Chartered Institute of Personnel and Development
DH	Department of Health
GP	general practitioner
IPO	input-process-output
IT	information technology
NHS	National Health Service
NHSME	National Health Service Management Executive

All web references in the following text were correct at the time of printing.

Preface

Whenever you talk to people using health and social services, they often assume that the different agencies and professions talk to each other regularly, actively share information and work closely together. Indeed, most people don't distinguish between 'health' and 'social care' at all – or between individual professions such as 'nursing', 'social work' or 'occupational therapy'. They simply have 'needs' that they want addressing in a professional and responsive manner – ideally by someone they know and trust. How the system is structured behind the scenes could not matter less.

And yet, people working in health and social care know that it *does* matter. None of us starts with a blank sheet of paper, and we all have to finds ways of working in a system that was not designed with integration in mind. As the books in this series explain, different parts of our health and social care services have evolved over time as largely separate entities, and policy-makers, managers and front-line practitioners trying to offer a joined-up service will typically face a series of practical, legal, financial and cultural barriers. This is often time-consuming and frustrating, and the end result for service users and their families often still does not feel very integrated (no matter how hard the professionals were working to try to produce a joint way forward). As one key commentator suggests, 'you can't integrate a square peg into a round hole' (Leutz, 1999, p 93).

When services aren't joined-up, it can result in poor outcomes for everybody – gaps, duplication and wasted time and resources. People using services frequently express amazement at the number of different people they have to tell their story to. Instinctively, it doesn't feel like a good use of their time or of the skilled professionals who are trying to help them. Often, one part of the system can't do something until they've had input from another part, and this can lead to all kinds of delays, inefficiencies and missed opportunities.

For staff, it can be surprisingly difficult to find enough time and space to gain a better understanding of how other agencies and professions operate, what they do, what priorities they have and what constraints they face. For someone who went into a caring profession to make a difference, there is nothing more dispiriting than knowing that someone needs a joined-up response but not knowing how to achieve it. In many situations, workers feel they are being asked to help people with complex needs, but with one hand constantly tied behind their back.

For the broader system, this state of affairs seems equally counter-productive. If support is delayed or isn't sufficiently joined-up, it can lead to needs going unmet and to people's health rapidly deteriorating. It then becomes even harder and even more expensive to intervene in a crisis – and this leaves less time and money for other people who are becoming unwell and need support (thus creating a vicious cycle). Poor communication, duplication and arguments over who should pay for what all lead to inefficiency, bad feeling and poor outcomes for people using services. In extreme cases, a lack of joint working can also culminate in very serious, tragic situations – such as a child death, a mental health homicide, the abuse of a person with learning difficulties or an older person dying at home alone (see Box 0.1 for but one high profile example). Here, partnership working is quite literally a matter of life and death, and failure to collaborate can have the most serious consequences for all involved.

Box 0.1: Partnership working as a matter of life or death

Following the tragic death of Peter Connelly (initially known as 'Baby P' in the press), Lord Laming (2009) was asked to produce a national review of progress since his initial investigation into the equally horrific death of Victoria Climbié in the same borough of Haringey (Laming, 2003). As the 2009 review observed (Laming, 2009, para 4.3):

> It is evident that the challenges of working across organisational boundaries continue to pose barriers in practice, and that cooperative efforts are often the first to suffer when services and individuals are under pressure. Examples of poor practice highlighted to this report include child protection conferences where not all the services involved in a child's life are present or able to give a view; or where one professional disagrees with a decision and their view is not explored in more detail; and repeated examples of professionals not receiving feedback on referrals. As a result of each of these failures, children or young people at risk of neglect or abuse will be exposed to greater danger. The referring professional may also be left with ongoing anxiety and concern about the child or young person. This needs to be addressed if all local services are to be effective in keeping children and young people safe.

For health and social care practitioners, if you are to make a positive and practical difference to service users and patients, most of the issues you face will involve working with other professions and other organisations. For public service managers, partnership working is likely to occupy an increasing amount of your time and budget, and arguably requires different skills and approaches to those prioritised in traditional single agency training and development courses. For social policy students and policy-makers, many of the issues you study and/or try to resolve inevitably involve multiple professions and multiple organisations. Put simply, people do not live their lives according to the categories we create in our welfare services – real-life problems are nearly always messier, more complex, harder to define and more difficult to resolve than this.

Policy context

In response, national and local policy increasingly calls for enhanced and more effective partnership working as a potential solution (see, for example, DH, 2013). While such calls for more joint working can be inconsistent, grudgingly made and/or overly aspirational, the fact remains that collaboration between different professions and different organisations is increasingly seen as the norm (rather than as an exception to the rule). This is exemplified in a previous Welsh policy paper, *The sustainable social services for Wales: A framework for action* (Welsh Assembly Government, 2011, p 11) that argued, 'We want to change the question from "how might we cooperate across boundaries?" to justifying why we are not.' With most new funding and most new policy initiatives, there is usually a requirement that local agencies work together to bid for new resources or to deliver the required service, and various Acts of Parliament place statutory duties of partnership on a range of public bodies. As an example of the growing importance of partnership working, in 1999 the word 'partnership' was recorded 6,197 times in official parliamentary records, compared to just 38 times in 1989 (Jupp, 2000, p 7). When we repeated this exercise for the first edition of this book, we found 17,912 parliamentary references to 'partnership' in 2006 alone (although this fell to 11,319 when removing references to legislation on civil partnerships that was being debated at the time). Since then, there have been two general elections/ new governments and a series of major spending cuts and pressures – arguably making joint working harder to achieve in practice, but even more important.

In 1998, the Department of Health issued a consultation document on future relationships between health and social care. Entitled

Partnership in action, the document proposed various ways of promoting more effective partnerships, basing these on a scathing but extremely accurate critique of single agency ways of working:

> All too often when people have complex needs spanning both health and social care good quality services are sacrificed for sterile arguments about boundaries. When this happens people, often the most vulnerable in our society ... and those who care for them find themselves in the no man's land between health and social services. This is not what people want or need. It places the needs of the organisation above the needs of the people they are there to serve. It is poor organisation, poor practice, poor use of taxpayers' money – it is unacceptable. (DH, 1998, p 30)

Whatever you might think about subsequent policy and practice, the fact that a government document sets out such a strongly worded statement of its beliefs and guiding principles is important. How to move from the rhetoric to reality is always the key challenge – but such quotes illustrate that partnership working is no longer an option (if it ever was), but core business. Under the coalition government (2010-15), this previous language shifted once again – and most recent policy refers to the importance of 'integrated care' (rather than 'partnerships' or 'collaboration'). As the coalition's NHS Future Forum (2012, p 3) argued:

> Integration is a vitally important aspect of the experience of health and social care for millions of people. It has perhaps the greatest relevance for the most vulnerable and those with the most complex and long-term needs. We have services to be proud of, and patients in England already receive some of the most joined-up services in the world. However, too many people fall through gaps between services as they traverse journeys of care which are often too difficult for them to navigate themselves. This lack of integration results

daily in delays and duplication, wasted opportunities and patient harm. It is time to "mind the gaps" and improve the experience and outcomes of care for people using our services.

While it is not always fully clear what a commitment to more integrated care might mean in practice (see below for further discussion), recent policy seems to be trying to achieve a number of different things, including:

- greater *vertical integration* between acute, community and primary care
- greater *horizontal integration* between community health and social care
- more effective joint working between *public health* and local government
- more effective partnerships between the *public, private and voluntary sectors*
- more *person-centred care*, with services that feel integrated to the patient.

In response to all this, the time feels right for a second edition of this book and of our 'Better partnership working' Series more generally. While our overall approach remains the same (see below for a summary of our aims and ethos), key changes to this edition include:

- updated references to current policy and practice
- the addition of more recent studies and broader literature
- a greater focus on 'integrated care' under the coalition government (2010-15) and the Conservative government of 2015-
- new reflective exercises and updated further reading/resources
- updated 'hot topics' (with a particular focus in some of the books in the series on the importance of working together during a time of austerity).

Aims and ethos

Against this background, this book (and the overall series of which it is part) provides an introduction to partnership working via a series of accessible 'how to' resources (see Box 0.2). Designed to be short and easy to use, they are nevertheless evidence-based and theoretically robust. A key aim is to provide *rigour and relevance* via books that:

- offer practical support to those working with other agencies and professions and to provide some helpful frameworks with which to make sense of the complexity that partnership working entails;
- summarise current policy and research in a detailed but accessible manner;
- provide practical but also evidence-based recommendations for policy and practice.

Box 0.2: The series at a glance

- *Partnership working in health and social care* (Jon Glasby and Helen Dickinson, 2nd edn)
- *Managing and leading in inter-agency settings* (Helen Dickinson and Gemma Carey, 2nd edn)
- *Interprofessional education and training* (John Carpenter and Helen Dickinson, 2nd edn)
- *Working in teams* (Kim Jelphs, Helen Dickinson and Robin Miller, 2nd edn)
- *Evaluating outcomes in health and social care* (Helen Dickinson and Janine O'Flynn, 2nd edn)

While each book is cross-referenced with others in the series, each is a standalone text with all you need to know as a student, practitioner, manager or policy-maker to make sense of the difficulties inherent in partnership working. In particular, the series aims to provide some practical examples to illustrate the more theoretical knowledge of social policy students, and some theoretical material to help make sense of the practical experiences and frustrations of front-line workers and managers.

Although there is a substantial literature on partnership working (see, for example, Hudson, 2000; Payne, 2000; Rummery and Glendinning, 2000; Balloch and Taylor, 2001; 6 et al, 2002; Glendinning et al, 2002; Sullivan and Skelcher, 2002; Barrett et al, 2005; Glasby and Dickinson, 2014a, for just some of many potential examples), most current books are either broad edited collections, very theoretical books that are inaccessible for students and practitioners, or texts focusing on partnership working for specific user groups. Where more practical, accessible and general texts exist, they typically lack any real depth or evidence base – in many ways, they are little more than partnership 'cookbooks' that give apparently simple instructions that are meant to lead to the perfect and desired outcome. In practice, anyone who has studied or worked in health and social care knows that partnership working can be both frustrating and messy – even if you follow the so-called 'rules', the end result is often hard to predict, ambiguous and likely to provoke different reactions from different agencies and professions. In contrast, this book series seeks to offer a more 'warts and all' approach to the topic, acknowledging the realities that practitioners, managers and policy-makers face in the real world.

Wherever possible, the series focuses on key concepts, themes and frameworks rather than on the specifics of current policy and organisational structures (which inevitably change frequently). As a result, the series will hopefully be of use to readers in all four countries of the UK as well as other national settings. That said, where structures and key policies have to be mentioned, they will typically be those in place in England.

While the focus of the series is on public sector health and social care, it is important to note from the outset that current policy and practice also emphasises a range of additional partnerships and relationships, including:

- broader partnerships (for example, with services such as transport and leisure in adult services and with education and youth justice in children's services);
- collaboration not just between services, but also between professionals and people who use services;
- relationships between the public, private and voluntary sectors.

As a result, many of the frameworks and concepts in each book may focus initially on public sector health and social care, but will also be relevant to a broader range of practitioners, students, services and service users.

Ultimately, the current emphasis on partnership working and on integration means that everything about public services – their organisation and culture, professional education and training, inspection and quality assurance – will have to change. Against this background, we hope that this series of books is a contribution, however small, to these changes.

Jon Glasby and Helen Dickinson
University of Birmingham and University of Melbourne
December 2015

1

What is teamworking and why does it matter?

Teams are an important component of everyday life. If you are employed it is likely that you sit in some form of team; if you are studying you will at some point engage in teamwork for a particular project or activity; and in your leisure time you may play in a sports team or support at least one team. Teamworking is an activity that most of us engage in on a regular basis without even consciously thinking about it. Teams can be incredibly important to us on a human level and contribute to our identity, wellbeing, sense of belonging and community. Similarly, in the context of public services, teams are thought to be important in terms of driving organisational and system performance.

At present, local health and social care communities are under significant pressure as challenges arising from the impacts of austerity measures combine with greater citizen expectations, the vestiges of repeated reorganisations of different government agencies and functions and changes to balances of professional power. Government and non-government organisations alike are tasked with achieving the holy trinity of doing more with fewer resources and in a more joined-up and user-centric way. Dealing with complex and cross-cutting issues while there is such turbulence in the system is no easy thing to achieve, and many individuals and organisations have sought to identify the means through which to improve the performance of their organisations and also the broader systems in which they are embedded.

At least part of the answer to this challenge is effective teamwork. As Glasby and Dickinson argue in the introductory book in this series (see *Partnership working in health and social care*, 2014a), it is not easy to make partnerships work. Although there are a range of frameworks and models available to aid collaborative working, in practice it is the human factor – the individuals and groups comprising the collaboration – that will ultimately make it a success (or not). At the core of the literature on teamworking is a focus on the human factor.

This book builds on a range of theories, models and research to demonstrate the benefits (and pitfalls) inherent in teamworking, and provides frameworks and practical advice on how teams and inter-agency teams may be made to function more effectively. This edition has been updated since the previous publication in a number of ways, drawing not only on new research evidence, but also on the outcomes of a series of different inquiries into incidents of poor quality care that we have seen emerge globally. In addition to updating the policy context, using more contemporary examples and incorporating global learning about teamworking, we have also sought out more tools and frameworks that can be used by professionals to improve teamwork in their organisations.

In coming to revise this text, one reflection we have as a team of authors is just how much new material has been published on the topic of teamworking across a range of different disciplines. We have sought to synthesise this material and from this extract the kinds of lessons and frameworks that will be of most use to those leading teams in the context of inter-agency working. This kind of activity is important because, although teams are viewed as crucial building blocks across a range of sectors, effective teams cannot be formed by simply grouping individuals together, even though this is often what happens in practice. In the same way that 'partnership' became a buzzword in the late 1990s and early 2000s, and 'community' and 'empowerment' were similarly popular in the 1980s, in recent years 'teams' and 'teamworking' have become catchphrases within the fields of management and organisational behaviour. Consequently it could be suggested that teams have become the (unspoken) core building blocks of many of the so-called 'fads' of modern management (for example, empowerment, business process re-engineering, quality services and management, and the learning organisation).

However, just because something is called a team does not mean that the predicted benefits will simply automatically flow from this arrangement or, indeed, that teamworking is the best way to bring about particular changes. In order to gain the full range of benefits that are associated with teamworking, relationships must be forged between team members, and between teams and the wider organisational environment. Research evidence shows a range of ways in which this process might be enhanced, and this is further explored in the following chapters, as are a series of lessons about what might hinder it. A number of mechanisms for more effective teamworking will likely be recognisable and seem, to some extent, intuitive to many of us. However, within the busy day-to-day world of service delivery, it is these basic building blocks that are all too often overlooked.

Despite criticisms that teamworking might be somewhat of a current fad, there is considerable and growing evidence that effective teamworking can create a significant impact on organisational performance (covered in more detail in Chapter 2). However, it is not just the potential for improvement that is driving this agenda – there are very practical ramifications when teamworking goes wrong. Box 1.1 illustrates the implications of effective and ineffective teamwork with case studies that most of us will be familiar with.

Box 1.1: Case examples of successful and unsuccessful teamworking

One example of the implications of ineffective teamworking that has received significant dissection and debate in the media is the US government's response to Hurricane Katrina, which hit New Orleans in August 2005. The storm following this weather event flooded New Orleans, and events that followed killed nearly 2,000 people and caused over US$100 billion in property damage. This was despite the fact that weather forecasters had warned the government about the approach of Katrina, and arrangements were in place for an emergency team to respond to this kind of incidence. In the formal report into the disaster response (United States House of Representatives, 2006) several reasons were given for the failure to respond, but key are the unfamiliarity of different agencies with their roles and responsibilities, and confusion over

3

assignments, deployments and the command structure. Communication broke down and key individuals and organisations did not speak to one another enough. Failure to take decisions meant that action was not taken on key issues. Overall, there was uncertainty about who was in charge, and red tape slowed down a number of response processes. Across the world we saw images in the media of the impacts of ineffective teamworking, where journalists were actually out on boats rescuing individuals, as they were the first to reach them.

If we compare this example to the Chilean mining disaster of 2010, we see a very different picture. In this case 33 miners were trapped below ground in the San Jose mine. For the first 17 days there was no contact with the miners, but even after contact was made, the team above ground were predicting that it could take them up to four months to release the miners. However, after just two-and-a-half months, all of the miners emerged. Urzua, the leader of the miners, had rallied the members around a clear goal (surviving), allocated roles linked to skill sets, collectively made decisions, and where issues arose, discussed which solutions were better suited to their end goal (Scandura and Sharif, 2013). The team on the surface also worked well together and, once in contact with the miners, collected appropriate information and used this to help the rescue effort. In this case we saw multiple teams working well individually and also collectively across teams. The organisation above ground worked well with the media to cover the incident in a positive way that would not hamper the rescue effort.

In both these cases serious disasters occurred that had the potential for significant loss of life. Yet in the latter example, clarity of goal, clear delineation of roles and good communication meant that teamwork ultimately had a positive impact. Unfortunately for the residents of New Orleans, the same could not be said, and a lack of coordination and communication led to the death and serious injury of many individuals and events that will have a lasting impact for many.

As these examples illustrate, teamworking does not just come about because we bring a group of people together, and we need to think carefully about how teamworking is supported. This book aims to support those who wish to create effective teams by setting out some of the kinds of factors that are important to consider. In the remainder of this chapter we consider a range of definitions and distinctions that are important to understand when thinking through the different types of teamworking mechanisms that might be necessary within inter-agency contexts. Although teamworking in collaborative settings often involves a much wider range of professional groups with different values, procedures and approaches than more traditional situations, there are certainly lessons from wider, more developed literatures that can inform these processes. The next section considers the relationship between teamworking and collaboration in more detail, before considering what it means to be an effective team, summarising the current UK policy context.

Relationship between teamworking and collaboration

One of the questions that we are often asked is what the difference is between *teamworking* and *collaborative working*. When we talk about collaborative working we are often talking about different professionals coming together to work towards particular ends – so this raises the question of whether collaboration is a different thing to teamworking. Inevitably the answer to this question is yes and no, and largely depends on how we use language. A fundamental principle of teamworking is that it involves collaborating with others; similarly, achieving inter-agency collaboration often involves teamworking. In driving improvement it seems that we need both collaborative working and teamworking.

One way to think about the difference between these two concepts is in terms of the contribution that these different literatures make. As Dickinson (2014) notes, the literature on collaboration has predominantly focused on the macro level, being largely concerned with the formal structures and mechanisms that might be used to bring about more joined-up services for users. The introductory book in this series by Glasby and Dickinson (2014a) provides a good account of this literature for those seeking to understand this in more detail. In addition to contributions around the macro level, there are a growing number of accounts that focus on individuals in front-line practice, and an account of this is provided in another book in this series, *Managing and leading in inter-agency settings*, by Dickinson and Carey (2016). The teamworking literature focuses on the level between formalised structures and individual practice, being concerned with the activities of groups of professionals. In this sense we can think of the contribution of the teamworking literature being at the meso level. If we wish to create effective collaborative working in practice, the reality is that we need to consider factors at all three levels, and it is possible that initiatives at one level may be undermined by those at another if they do not effectively align.

It is sometimes argued that teamworking can be more difficult in inter-agency settings. A classic description of this comes from the Audit Commission (1992, p 20):

> Separate lines of control, different payment systems leading to suspicion over motives, diverse objectives, professional barriers and perceived inequalities in status, all play a part in limiting the potential of multiprofessional, multiagency teamwork. These undercurrents often lead to a rigidity within teams with members adhering to narrow definitions of their role preventing the creation of flexible responses required to meet the variety of human need presented ... for those working under such circumstances efficient teamwork remains elusive.

While undoubtedly these are challenges, we argue that many of these sorts of characteristics are also present in 'traditionally' structured settings (for example, hospitals). In thinking about what sorts of literatures to draw on for this book, we chose to be inclusive and not simply focus on research and evidence derived from inter-agency settings. This has proved to be both a blessing and a curse given that this literature is huge. We tried to select the most appropriate lessons for health and social care collaborations, but inevitably there are trade-offs in terms of what has been included and what we have had to omit. We could have filled this book at least ten times over with possible examples and frameworks, so wherever possible, we have tried to signpost other useful sources that students and practitioners will be able to pursue further.

What do we mean by teams and teamworking?

When reading academic research, one of the challenges is getting to grips with a set of highly specialised terminology that may be unfamiliar unless you have a detailed knowledge of this area. For many individuals reading the teamworking literature, this might not be a problem given that we have noted the familiarity of the concepts of 'teams' and 'teamworking'. However, the ubiquity of the terminology surrounding teamworking is in some ways a challenge in itself. Much as the terminology surrounding collaboration has been used to refer to a wide range of different sorts of working arrangements, so, too, has the concept of a team: using terminology to refer to lots of different things can lead to the loss of any original power it might have had. If we use the term 'team' to refer to everything, then there is a risk that this widespread use might fuel cynicism about these concepts, and front-line practitioners might be reluctant to engage with these agendas because they have seen this before and nothing significant seems to have changed.

We believe that *real* teams (see Chapter 2 for a discussion of 'real' versus 'pseudo' teams) are important in delivering high quality services, and it follows that we think it important to be clear about language. In the example of Hurricane Katrina, for example, there was a team in place, but a lack of clarity over roles and responsibilities meant that it did not act as a *real* team in practice. In this section we explore the research literature in terms of how it specifically defines different terms, and establish meanings that we use throughout this book.

In Box 1.2 we set out some of the different definitions of teams and teamworking that we find in the literature. As these illustrate, there is some significant difference in how these terms are used. What is considered a team within a hospital is likely to differ to that in a primary care, mental health or respite care setting. Whether teams are temporary or permanent, where their members are from, whether membership is voluntary, what tasks the team is supposed to achieve and the level of specialised skills the team requires – all are important markers of distinction between teams. As Salas and colleagues (2000, p 343) note, 'all teams are not equal', and Appelbaum and Batt (1994) suggest that the failure to differentiate between different forms of teamworking (see Box 1.3) is partly why research has found the effects of teamworking to be inconsistent. Just as it is important for researchers to make sure that they are comparing the same things when talking about teams, a key issue for students and front-line workers when using the terms 'team' and 'teamworking' is to check out that all partners understand the same thing by these terms.

Although teams are a relatively modern phenomenon, there is a long and established tradition of research into groups. The groups literature is incredibly diverse in nature, having roots in multiple different disciplines, fields of research and organisational settings. In contemporary studies it is generally acknowledged that teams and groups are different entities (although this may only be a degree of difference). Size is sometimes used as a differentiator here. Mueller et al (2000) suggest that a team is composed of between 3 and 15 members, while Belbin (2000) states that the maximum size for a team is no more than 6 to 8. As a general rule, groups tend to be larger in size than teams, although this is by no means definitive.

Box 1.2: Helpful definitions

Drawing on a large review of the commercial sector literature, Cohen and Bailey (1997, p 241) describe a team as:

> ... a collection of individuals who are interdependent in their tasks, who share responsibility for outcomes, who see themselves and who are seen by others as an intact social entity embedded in one or more larger social systems (for example, business unit or the corporation) and who manage their relationship across organisational boundaries.

Hawkins and his colleagues (2014) at a Bath consultancy group extended a very well known and respected definition of a team from Katzenbach and Smith (1993, p 35), to describe a team as:

> A small number of people with complementary skills who are committed to a common purpose, set of performance goals and shared approach, for which they hold themselves mutually accountable. The common goal needs to include ways of effectively meeting and communicating that raise morale and alignment, effectively engaging with all the team's key stakeholder groups, and ways that individuals and that team can continually learn and develop.

West and colleagues (1998) suggest three criteria for a group to be considered a team: the group needs to have a defined organisational function and identity; the group must possess shared objectives or goals; and the team members must have interdependent roles.

In Box 1.3 we set out a number of different sorts of teams and groups as a way to illustrate these definitional points. As you examine these, it is also important to note that individuals may work in more than one type of team. This can often make for incredibly complex service delivery contexts.

Box 1.3: Different types of teams and groups and means of collaboration

There is a range of different types of teams that may be found within health and social care organisations. Here is an overview of the more common ways they can be classified, although it is by no means exhaustive.

Work undertaken

Sundstrom (1999) identified six types of teams, distinguished by the type of work they do: production; service; management; project; action/performing; and parallel teams. These teams also differ in terms of at least four further factors: level of authority within the wider organisation; time until the team is disbanded; degree of specialisation, independence and autonomy in relation to other teams; and the degree to which they are interdependent within the team as well as with forces outside the team.

Lean teams are designed around particular processes and have complete responsibility for identifying problems, creating solutions and implementing actions to make processes as efficient and effective as possible (see, for example, Burgess and Radnor, 2013; Morrow et al, 2014).

Location of members

Virtual teams (or geographically dispersed teams) are a group of individuals who work across time, space and organisational boundaries, often using information technology (IT) to strengthen links. These are becoming an increasingly important feature of many contemporary organisations. Co-located teams, on the other hand, are those that share a physical space such as an office or service base.

Degree of autonomy

Self-directed or *self-managed teams* have full responsibility for the product or service that they produce, including the management of that process. The point of difference between these two types is that self-directed teams identify the goal that they are aiming to achieve.

Due to the recognition that better partnership between organisations will result in closed integration of services as a means to improve outcomes, there is a particular interest in teams involving a diversity of roles and members drawn from different organisations. There are a whole set of terms commonly applied to such teams (see Box 1.4).

Box 1.4: Teams and integration

- *Multiprofessional:* practitioners who share the same professional background who practice within two or more different specialities or branches working side by side. This term is often used interchangeably, and for many it is about a range of professionals working together (or not).
- *Multidisciplinary:* practitioners from two or more different disciplines working side by side.
- *Multiagency:* practitioners from two or more different agencies working side by side. *Note:* The 'multi-' prefix implies that members of that group are not necessarily collaborating and might simply be working side by side, in parallel, or sequentially towards a common problem. However, when the term 'team' is used as a suffix, it should imply that members are collaborating and working towards shared objectives.
- *Interprofessional:* practitioners who share the same professional background and practice within two or more different specialities or branches working together.
- *Interdisciplinary:* practitioners from two or more different disciplines working together.
- *Inter-agency:* practitioners from two or more different agencies working together. *Note:* The 'inter-' prefix denotes that there are definite interactions between the members and there is active joint collaboration towards a problem, although members may not be approaching it from the same conceptual frameworks. The 'inter-' prefix further tends to denote a greater propensity for team members to be willing to work across boundaries, which multiprofessional teams may be less willing to do. Again, whether the suffix 'team' or 'working'

is used should indicate whether this collaboration is towards a specific end the members are jointly accountable for achieving.

- *Transdisciplinary:* members transcend their separate, conceptual and methodological orientations to overcome the disciplinary bounds that are present in multidisciplinary and interdisciplinary teams. Some commentators suggest that this is the only way to produce a truly integrated response to issues, although others have highlighted the dangers that might result from working in this way (considered further in Chapter 2).

McIntyre and Salas (1995) rather simplistically describe teamwork and teamworking as what a team does when it behaves as a team. This statement is a clear tautology, but it does draw attention to the fact that teamworking is effectively a team in action. There is a tendency to think of teams as internal units (that is, not linked into wider systems), which, according to McIntyre and Salas' description, would mean that teamworking is simply an expression of those internal processes. However, as the Chilean mining example set out in Box 1.1 illustrates, teamworking often involves the collaboration of teams, as well as simply individuals.

One metaphor that usefully describes the way teams have tended to operate in health and social care is as a castle, surrounded by a moat. Teams tend to be created and viewed as independent units, and where these prove successful, there is a risk that they are left to operate alone fairly autonomously. In terms of our metaphor, the castle may have its doors open and the drawbridge lowered, but members may not actually seek to enter or leave its confines. Conversely, when times are difficult there is a tendency for teams to pull up their drawbridge and to concentrate solely on internal issues. Recent experience of austerity and associated cuts to public sector budgets has arguably perpetuated some of this behaviour. Yet, in order for the whole system to operate effectively, teams must interact with each other and the wider environment. Teams must increasingly try to lower their drawbridges and operate beyond the confines of the 'castle'; they cannot operate autonomously from the rest of the system.

Teamworking, then, to some extent, is about a manifestation of teams working together, but importantly it is also about how teams relate to wider systems. The danger of teams operating in isolation is soberly highlighted by what is called the 'Nut Island effect' (Levy, 2001). In this case a committed, initially well-performing team was able to hide problems from the organisation that eventually led to a major disaster in a sewage treatment plant. The organisation gave a high degree of independence to the team as it had previously performed well, but this lack of wider linkages may have ultimately contributed to its failure, which had much wider implications than for the team alone.

So far we have provided an overview of the different definitions that tend to be associated with teams and teamworking, and suggested that when using these terms all partners should make sure that they understand the same things. One way of doing this within a collaborative setting is by using a descriptor that outlines the range of professionals the team is composed of, and the degree of collaboration between the members (Box 1.3 illustrates some of these terms). There are important distinctions between many of these terms, but they are often used interchangeably within the literature. Miller and colleagues (2001) note that notions of multidisciplinary or multiprofessional teams should not be confused with a group of professionals who work independently, but who happen to liaise with one another over a period of time. There are specific criteria that teams must meet to be considered so, and we need to be careful about how we demarcate teams in practice. If teams are misnamed, this could potentially have a significant impact: confusion over terms may mean that team members become unclear as to the nature of the team, as may supporting organisations. This terminology matters as we expect different things from different kinds of teams, and they require different forms of support.

Why does teamworking matter?

In the complex world of health and social care, it is unlikely that one individual will have the skills to fulfil all tasks. Teams are helpful because they have greater reach than individuals acting alone. As such, teamworking has been seen as a potential solution to any number of difficulties and complexities that organisations from a range of different sectors are currently facing. As organisations have become larger and more complex in structural terms, it has become ever more important that people work together in coordinated ways to achieve the overarching aims of their organisation. Organisations are now increasingly required to build in flexibility and to be more agile in order to be successful, and teamworking is seen as the most effective way of achieving this (Macy and Izumi, 1993; Appelbaum and Batt, 1994).

Often the principle motivation for organisations implementing teamworking is a belief that it will enhance their organisation's performance (Parker and Bradley, 2000). In Chapter 2 we provide an overview of a number of studies that have examined the link between teamworking and performance. In the context of health and social care, there is some evidence that teams that work together produce better outcomes for service users, staff members and the organisation (see, for example, O'Leary et al, 2012; West et al, 2013; Prades et al, 2015). Box 1.5 presents some of the positive impacts that teamwork is thought to be able to achieve. However, we must be cautious and not rush headlong into thinking that teamworking is the solution to everything (and there are clearly parallels here with the concept of collaborative working itself): teams take many different forms and will not necessarily deliver all (or any) of these suggested impacts. It is important that we unravel the causal chains involved in these processes so we can be clearer about what sorts of teams are able to bring about what sorts of effects and within which contexts.

Box 1.5: Why work in teams?

Mohrman et al (1995) set out a number of reasons why organisations might implement teamworking:

- Because of the need for consistency between organisational environment, strategy and design, teams are the best way to enact the strategy of organisations.
- Teams enable organisations to speedily develop and deliver services cost-effectively, while retaining high quality.
- Teams enable organisations to learn (and retain learning) more effectively.
- Cross-functional teams promote improved quality of services.
- Cross-functional teams can undertake effective process re-engineering.
- Time is saved if activities, formerly performed sequentially by individuals, can be performed concurrently by people working in teams.
- Innovation is promoted within team-based organisations because of cross-fertilisation of ideas.
- Flat organisations can be monitored, coordinated and directed more effectively if the functional unit is the team rather than the individual.
- As organisations have grown more complex, so, too, have their information-processing requirements; teams can integrate and link in ways individuals cannot.

Cohen and Bailey (1997, p 243) suggest three major dimensions of effectiveness that result from teamworking: performance effectiveness assessed in terms of quantity and quality of outputs (in health and social care collaboration this is likely to relate to service user outcomes and satisfaction, quality of care and safety); member attitudes; and behavioural outcomes. These different levels are interesting as Parker and Bradley (2000, p 24) note that employee satisfaction has been demonstrated to link to organisational performance, and those companies with high employee satisfaction have been shown to demonstrate better financial performance. Unhappy employees are more likely to be stressed, be absent from work and less likely to continue to work for a company.

Teamwork, therefore, might not only be beneficial in terms of a direct link to organisational performance, but could also create more satisfied staff members, who are more productive, less likely to be absent and more likely to enhance organisational performance. In this way, effective teamworking is thought to be able to trigger a kind of virtuous chain of events, where feedback enhances both individual and organisational performance (see Figure 1.1). Similarly, however, the converse is also thought to be true; ineffective teamworking might lead to lower staff satisfaction, negative behaviours and an inability to attract new quality staff members that might have a negative impact on organisational performance, which subsequently feeds back into team morale.

There is another factor that is missing from Figure 1.1, which will become increasingly important for providers and commissioners of services alike. If teamworking is effective within provider services, this could potentially increase a commissioning organisation's confidence in that service, and increase the possibility of that team being re-

Figure 1.1: Effective teamworking and feedback processes

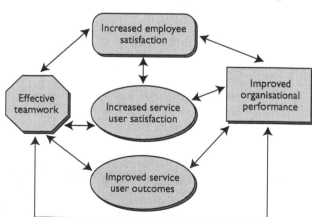

commissioned for a present or extended service or being awarded more autonomy. In a context that is still feeling the effects of a number of care scandals, there is more than ever a focus on the need to commission quality services effectively and safely. Therefore, commissioners will need to have an increasing interest in how care is delivered, and a key question in the future may relate to the degree to which organisations support teamworking.

Box 1.6 illustrates an example of an effective health and social care team and the impacts that this produced. Essentially this illustrates a number of the effects suggested in Figure 1.1 in practice.

Box 1.6: Example of team effectiveness

The Child and Adolescent Mental Health Services (CAMHS) Transformation Team is an inter-agency team, consisting of two CAMHS teams, a community paediatric team, a children's learning disability team, a children's commissioning team and voluntary sector teams along with children and young people. The team is working together in transforming emotional wellbeing services for children and young people, breaking down professional barriers and seeking creative alternative models to improve outcomes for young people. The team has a shared vision to transform mental health services for children and young people, and recognises that improving outcomes is dependent on working collaboratively across organisational boundaries. The team is committed to designing services around children and young people (not professionals and agencies), and not getting tied up in organisational limits and/or competitive practice. Each partner has committed financial or other resources to support this service transformation.

New parenting services established by the transformation team are demonstrating significant improved outcomes for families. One parent recently shared her experience of the parenting group at the trust's service user and carer celebration day. The teams are engaging with children and young people to redesign services. One of the service users recently presented at the national participation conference and was an award winner at the trust's service user and carer awards.

The team is using a range of approaches to increase young people's participation in the service. Examples include a participation day facilitated by young people, working with Arts for Health in art-based activities for participation, and running local parenting and young people's groups. Increasing young people's participation is, in turn, supporting a more creative approach to service delivery that doesn't rely on additional funding or resources, including annual emotional health checks for young people, young people facilitating support groups and a CAMHS website designed by young people.

Source: Provided by Jennie Collier (Head of Operations, Specialist and Family Services Directorate, South Staffordshire and Shropshire Healthcare NHS Foundation Trust)

Given the range of potential positive impacts teamworking is thought to be able to produce, health and social care workers are continually exhorted to work together to develop multidisciplinary teams and integrate services. Yet the degree to which these positives are empirically demonstrated is to some degree questionable (and is explored further in Chapters 2 and 3). Allen and Hecht (2004) suggest that a group of individuals working together under the title of a team do not necessarily achieve more than could be achieved by a group of competent individuals working alone, and that evidence shows that it is the psychological benefits or the 'romance of teams' that makes people think that their team is performing better. Furthermore, as previously demonstrated, not all teams are equal, and these potential benefits should be treated with healthy scepticism. Simply describing a group of individuals as a team will not guarantee that the benefits outlined in Figure 1.1 and Box 1.6 will automatically be experienced. Care must be taken to ensure that appropriate structures, procedures, senior leadership commitment, development and training opportunities are in place to get the most from teams.

Chapters 2 and 3 present a range of lessons from research (from both health and social care collaborations and wider relevant literatures) that suggest how effective teams may be formed and sustained. However, before this, the following section briefly considers the health and social care policy context to determine how the present onus on teamworking has developed over time.

Policy context

One of the ironies of the health and social care arena over the past quarter of a century has been that just as the concept of the 'whole patient' was being (re)-discovered through more modern perspectives of public health (acknowledging economic and sociocultural determinants of health; for further discussion see Baggott, 2010), the professions of health and social care have become ever more specialised and narrowly focused. Since the turn of the last century, generalist workers have been progressively replaced by a div rse range of occupations and specialists who are focused on particular fields of work, problem areas, processes or client groups. With rapidly advancing knowledge and changing technologies, professionals have become ever more specialised into specific areas.

In practice this shift can be perceived as positive – professionals have a much more detailed understanding of a certain problem or issue – but this can prove problematic in that it is unlikely that a single person can have exhaustive knowledge of their entire profession (or, indeed, other professions). Increased professional specialisation has led to the internal fragmentation of health and social care organisations, requiring professionals to work more closely and with a wider range of colleagues internally within their organisations. Over this period there has also been growing recognition that individuals often have multifactorial problems, which a single agency alone cannot solve, and which requires the input of multiple agencies. That is, while agencies are becoming increasingly internally specialised, requiring professional groups to work together, they are also being called on to work with outside agencies to provide services around the needs of individuals. Consequently, no one professional is likely to be able to provide all the support and assistance that an individual with chronic or complex needs requires, and we are starting to see expansive care pathways emerging for many conditions. Increasingly, the implication is that each profession and expert system is necessarily required to overlap with others. Teamworking has been seen as one way to work more effectively over both these internal and external boundaries.

As a result of these pressures, since the early 1970s we have started to see reference to entities such as primary care teams (BMA, 1974), community mental health teams (DH, 2002), intermediate care teams (DH, 2000) and any other number of teams organised around specific conditions or client groups. Not only are these teams thought to simplify 'patient journeys' and move towards the more seamless delivery of care, but also to reduce duplication, cut costs and potentially increase the productivity of the system. As one NHS Management Executive (NHSME, 1993) report suggests:

> The best and most cost-effective outcomes for patients and clients are achieved when professionals work together, learn together, engage in clinical audit of outcomes together, and generate innovation to ensure progress in practice and service.

Indeed, *The NHS Plan* (DH, 2000) went as far as to suggest that poor teamworking was one of the reasons why the NHS had failed to deliver on healthcare priorities in the past. This document claimed that the NHS was a '1940s system operating in a 21st-century world', which had failed due to its 'old-fashioned demarcations between staff and barriers between services' (DH, 2000, p 10). This analysis suggests that somehow working in teams can compensate for the limitations of current organisational structures, and reduce the irritations that these cause within the everyday work of staff members. However, successive reform processes have struggled to make this a reality in the context of health and social care. Aims and objectives for teams often remain more rhetoric than reality; in practice, effective teamworking often remains more aspirational and idealised than realised.

One of the difficulties in trying to summarise the policy context in respect to teamworking is that so many different areas of policy have an impact on teams and teamworking. Added to this, political devolution has meant that we have started to see quite different policies develop across the four countries of the UK. Health and social care communities have recently undergone, and are undergoing, some fairly fundamental changes in terms of their structures and configurations, all of which have had, and are having, impacts on the employment conditions and allegiances of staff members. Over the past 15 years or so we have witnessed a more profound split in terms of the commissioners and providers of services, diversification of provision (in health and social care), a rise in service user control (through mechanisms such as individual funding) and in England, the transfer of public health responsibilities from the NHS to local governments. Not only do such structural changes disrupt existing relationships between individuals and agencies, but they also fundamentally alter the compositions of traditional teams, and these have real impacts on the ways in which they are able to work together.

Yet structures are just one thing that has an impact on teams. The health and social care workforce is changing significantly with ongoing professionalisation and educational reforms, in addition to the influx of a number of overseas professionals, but also significant reductions in some areas of the workforce as austerity pressures bite. It seems unlikely, however, that the pace of change will slow. Days of stability for health and social care organisations seem to be a thing of the past, and increasingly it will be up to individuals and teams to make sense of this context and to lead through change. These changes clearly have important implications for teamworking, and individuals may find themselves working with people from a wider range of sectors and backgrounds than ever before.

Reflective exercises

1. Make a list of teams that you have encountered recently, both in your professional and personal life. Looking at the different definitions of teams set out in this chapter, how would you categorise these?

2. Ask a colleague or friend how they would define teams/teamworking. How does this compare to your understanding?

3. What do you think are the key things that make a 'real' team, and how are these different to other teams?

4. Have any of the teams you thought about in response to question 1 produced any of the positive effects outlined in this chapter that teamworking is thought to be able to achieve? Were there any negative impacts?

5. Think about a time where you have been part of an effective team. What did this feel like? What did you enjoy, and how might you be able to recreate this within another team setting?

Further reading and resources

There are a range of different websites and books that include introductory material about teams and teamworking, and examples of effective and ineffective teams. We include a selection of these below, and others are also referred to over the course of the text.

- Katzenbach and Smith's (1993) *The wisdom of teams* is a definitive work on creating high performance teams. It uses a number of cases and testimonials to illustrate successful and unsuccessful teamworking.
- Lencioni's (2012) *The advantage* is written by a *New York Times* bestselling author with a number of stories, tips and anecdotes from consulting to some of the top firms in the US.
- Pritchard and Eliot's (2012) *Help the helper* draws on lessons from top sports coaches to apply to organisations in order to create high quality supportive teamwork.
- The *Harvard Business Review*'s (2011) *Building better teams* includes a collection of papers on teamworking.
- See also West and Markiewicz's (2006) *The effective partnership working inventory*.
- A selection of different links to teamwork resources can be found at: http://reviewing.co.uk/toolkit/teams-and-teamwork.htm
- The University of Queensland has a video about team working in healthcare demonstrating a student learning exercise around a patient with complex needs: www.youtube.com/watch?v=qdxMANtPlhw
- The Canadian Foundation for Healthcare Improvement has a video describing the introduction of an interprofessional model of patient care: www.youtube.com/watch?v=syid_AAQqRo

2

What does research tell us?

As we saw in the last chapter, various claims have been made concerning the impacts that effective teamworking may have on both individuals and organisations, but similarly there are several reports where these assumed benefits have not always been fully realised. As Salas et al (2000, p 340) note, 'many organisations have, in the past, assumed that a team is a mere collection of individuals and, as such, assumed that merely putting members together would result in effective performance, but this is not true.' While there is a range of potential mitigating factors that might blunt the impact of teamworking, some commentators have also questioned the degree to which these presumed benefits have been demonstrated within a health and social care context. Zwarenstein and Reeves (2000, p 1022) describe this context as replete with rhetoric about the value of teamworking, but a lack of evidence to support the notion that it is necessarily a 'good thing' – hence their conclusion, 'what's so great about collaboration?'

In this chapter we consider the extent to which the aspirations of teamworking set out in Chapter 1 are reflected in the research evidence. As well as considering the findings of teams in health and social care in general, we focus in particular on the research evidence regarding teams in which professionals and practitioners from different disciplines and/or organisations work together. Increasingly professionals and practitioners are formally situated within teams that require interdisciplinary collaboration, and indeed, for many (for example, surgical teams), this has traditionally been the case. Not all teams in health and social care will involve different disciplines working together as a unified unit (for example, some health visitor, social work and domiciliary care teams). That said, most, if not all, of these 'uni-disciplinary' settings will involve staff undertaking different roles to the key profession such as nursing assistant or administration support, and there is still a need for these functions to work together successfully across health and social care systems. The key difference with the interdisciplinary teams that is our focus here is that in uni-disciplinary teams one discipline has the lead status with team functioning based around their dominant view. In interdisciplinary teams such an obvious hierarchy is generally not present, as their raison d'être is predicated on the creative tension and shared contributions of their diverse members.

In preparing this chapter we analysed literature reviews that included over 300 studies of teamworking in interdisciplinary settings. These included studies from different sectors (for example, acute, community, primary), organisational partnerships (for example, health-health and health-social care) and patient populations (for example, cancer, mental health, trauma). The large number of studies included highlights that interdisciplinary teamwork is an area of practice that has received a considerable level of research interest. That said, there are settings, population groups and professional groups in which such teams remain less investigated. At present acute hospitals (in particular, cancer services and emergency departments), general practice (in particular, joint working between general practitioners [GPs] and nurses) and mental health teams have received most attention.

As healthcare systems look to support more preventative services, within community rather than hospital settings, there needs to be further research around the teams that will need to be central to new and developing models of care – for example, primary care teams that include pharmacy and social work along with nursing and medicine, and preventative or rehabilitative teams that engage workers from the voluntary and community sector as well statutory health and social care. The continued problem of abuse of vulnerable adults and children would suggest that safeguarding teams require further exploration. There also remains little evidence of the potential economic benefits of 'real' rather than 'pseudo' teams (teams masquerading as well-functioning teams but lacking all the necessary characteristics – a point we return to later in this chapter). This evidence will be necessary not just so that we know what good teamworking looks like in these settings, but also to help in making the case for resource expenditure on team development in a context of extreme fiscal constraint.

This chapter is made up of two main sections. The first considers evidence regarding the impacts of teamworking and is arranged into three sub-themes – outcomes for service users, the experience of professionals and practitioners who work within teams (as their wellbeing and commitment is a key factor to effective delivery), and economic benefits (as using finances efficiently becomes increasingly important due to raised demands outweighing additional resources). The second section turns to the 'enablers' of teamworking, and is structured around inputs and processes. Table 2.1 summarises the evidence from key studies relating to teamworking.

What is the evidence about the impacts of teamworking?

Outcomes for service users

Mirroring much of the research regarding integrated care and partnerships (see Glasby and Dickinson, 2014b), team-based studies have more commonly reported on findings regarding difference in organisational functioning or processes within teams than any other factors. The evidence regarding outcomes for service users or economic benefits is typically described as being inconclusive or unsubstantial. However, as with the broader theme of collaboration, this may in part result from the difficulties that are inherent in evaluating inter-agency teamworking, given different objectives for teams, variations in local contexts and cultures as well as the variety of different theories and methods that have been used in research (see Dickinson and O'Flynn, 2016). Despite these evaluative difficulties, there is a decent body of evidence that suggests that good teamworking can lead to more effective outcomes for patients and service users (Richter et al, 2011).

Some of the most famous work is that of West et al (for example, 2002, 2013), looking at effective teamworking in the English NHS, and in particular, its connection with the way staff are managed, supported and organised. They found that there was a strong relationship between successful implementation of key human resource practices and a reduction in mortality rates, with teamworking being one of the three interventions with the strongest association. In hospitals in which 60% of staff members reported working in formal teams, mortality was 5% below the expected level (West et al, 2002), and that of other factors were consistent: a 5% increase in staff working in well-structured teams would lead to a 3.6% lower mortality rate (West et al, 2013). Patient satisfaction and overall rating of the care received is also shown to be higher within organisations that have a stronger culture of teamworking (O'Leary et al, 2012).

Such positive findings have also been reported in relation to interdisciplinary teams with a variety of settings and services. For example, Prades et al (2015) found that 100% of studies of interdisciplinary teams in cancer care that explored patient outcomes reported positive impacts, including increased rates of survival, improved patient satisfaction and better diagnosis and/or treatment planning. Franx et al (2008) highlight the benefits of assertive community treatment teams, where professionals work intensively and holistically with people with severe mental health problems who have a history of disengaging with services and have required numerous hospital admissions in the past. The teams are available on a 24-hour, seven days a week basis, with smaller caseloads than would generally be the case within community services.

Positive impacts include avoiding periods of hospitalisation (including those in which the person is detained against their will), an improved social situation such as stability of accommodation, and a reduction in the severity of people's symptoms. The organisational/ partnership context in which these teams are operating appears to have an influence on the outcomes for patients and service users. For example, in the US there are several studies of older people accessing the Veterans Administration system that report improved mental health, higher functional status, reduced dependency, lowered mortality and better health-related quality of life in services centred on multidisciplinary teams than those that took a more fragmented sequential approach. Interestingly these positive benefits were not replicated in other organisational contexts, despite similar models of team-based care (Lemieux-Charles and McGuire, 2006).

Another way of understanding outcomes for service users is to gain their views of the support that they have received. The evidence here is more mixed in relation to interdisciplinary teams, with some studies reporting that such teams led to services being more responsive to the needs of service users, and others reporting that the experience of service users was, in fact, poor (Maslin-Prothero and Bannion, 2010). Key issues highlighted in the latter were difficulties in gaining access to services, lack of clarity regarding what they were entitled to, and being treated insensitively when they were refused services. O'Driscoll et al (2014) compared the experiences of service users of teams for people with physical disabilities and teams for people with mental health problems. Those accessing physical disability services reported that they experienced high quality care and good communication, and trusted the advice and decisions of clinicians. Mental health service users, however, had quite a different view, and expressed frustration and disagreement with the decisions made by interdisciplinary teams and their apparent unwillingness to listen to the service user's perspective and/or to be challenged. This may be due to a shared or contrasting inherent belief about the nature of illnesses between professionals and service users and/or the respective levels of resources available in the service areas. These very different experiences of service users highlight that creating a structure around such teams will not, by itself, guarantee that the experience of those accessing them will necessarily be better. It is therefore vital that the focus of teams is on those that they support, rather than enforcing organisational criteria and processes, and that relevant data is gathered to enable teams to understand the impacts on the populations that they serve.

Table 2.1: Summary of evidence from key studies

Focus	Methods	Findings	Reference
Multidisciplinary teamworking in the NHS	Surveys completed by around 400 primary, community or secondary healthcare teams and in-depth qualitative work with a sub-sample of teams	Multidisciplinary teams with clear objectives, positive leadership and appropriate communication result in higher levels of participation, greater commitment to quality, and more effective and innovative practice. Team members within effective teams experience better wellbeing, and there is lower turnover of staff. Sufficient professional diversity is another key enabler	Borrill et al (2001)
Integration of social care staff within community mental health teams	National survey of mental health trusts, staff survey in four locations selected purposely for their differently constituted teams and interviews with service users	Staff perception that integrated teamworking is supported through better management, diversity of professions, social support and fewer job demands. Overall job satisfaction of team members is associated with the level of choice experienced by users, and their satisfaction with these choices (although the study notes the need for further exploration of outcomes)	Huxley et al (2011)
Principle factors that enable multiprofessional teamworking to improve care for service users	Survey of 135 teams in 11 NHS trusts and in-depth ethnographic studies of 19 teams involved in the survey	Team effectiveness factors included encouragement for innovation, team participation in decision-making, trust between members, leadership, skill mix and absence of conflict. Wider contextual factors included organisational support, sufficiency of resources (in particular, staff) and external targets. Effective teams promoted engagement with service users and carers, and sought partnerships with other teams and services	West et al (2012)
Staff engagement and its relationship with organisational performance	Analysis of NHS staff survey and other data sets between 2006 and 2009	Good management that encourages engagement is significantly associated with patient satisfaction, patient mortality and infection rates, as well as staff absenteeism and turnover. Ensuring that teams have clear objectives and teamworking is effective are key factors in developing a culture of engagement	West et al (2013)

Experience of professionals and practitioners

People deliver the majority of health and social care services, so improving the effectiveness of these services is closely connected with maintaining a committed and skilled workforce. For many organisations working in this sector, there is also recognition that staff members are individuals in their own right, and their wellbeing is also important. Borrill and colleagues (2001) found that those individuals working in clearly defined secondary care teams had lower levels of stress than those not working in teams or working in loose groupings. The researchers suggest that teamworking provides more social support and role clarity to individuals than those not working within teams or those who are only quasi-members. Borrill et al (2001, p 162) go on to suggest that these factors account for the difference in stress levels between membership types, suggesting, 'it is as though, by working in a team, team members achieve a shared level of self-sufficiency that buffers team members from the inadequacies of their organisations.' Job satisfaction is also promoted within interdisciplinary teams due to better communication and cooperation with other professions and agencies, leading to perceived improvements in responsiveness to patients and service users (Maslin-Prothero and Bennion, 2010; Prades et al, 2015).

Box 2.1 illustrates the experiences of professionals from around the world working in such teams with positive benefits including reduction in stress, opportunities for reflective practice, reduction in risk and the satisfaction of being part of a high-performing service (Reeves et al, 2011). However, there is a caveat to this evidence; these impacts were only shown to result where there were *real* interdependencies and social support between team members. Drawing again on the annual English NHS staff survey, West et al (2013) highlight that working in well-structured teams is correlated with lower staff absenteeism, reduced staff turnover and increased levels of engagement. Good engagement of staff with their organisation has been shown to be increase productivity, reduce errors and improve the wellbeing of employees (Ellins and Ham, 2009).

Box 2.1: International experiences of working within interdisciplinary teams

'There's the knowledge that the patient has received the best care possible, and that during the surgery the team worked cohesively together – it's "poetry in motion" to watch.' (nurse from Australia)

'Efficiency and competency in practice is another by-product of an interdisciplinary team. Workload sharing and stress reduction is also a significant factor in teamwork.' (occupational therapist from Canada)

'… interdisciplinary teamwork also gives an opportunity to coordinate efforts and have mutual reflections on how to understand the service user's situation which can be very complex.' (social worker from Norway)

'Working in a team and looking after very disturbed, difficult, aggressive and sometimes violent people, the teamworking approach made the area safe for service users and staff.' (mental health practitioner from the UK)

Source: Reeves et al (2011, pp 30-2)

Thus, teamworking is thought to have a significant effect on members, providing both social support and clarity around their role and tasks. All these aspects reduce uncertainty and stress, and increase satisfaction. Where individuals fail to understand their role, this is one of the biggest causes of stress within the workplace. Box 2.2 illustrates an example of a rehabilitation team where staff members did not fully understand either their own roles or the roles of their colleagues, and the implications this had.

Box 2.2: Implications of teams without clarity of vision or roles

Members of a newly established multidisciplinary rehabilitation team were struggling to work together effectively. The atmosphere was poor, relationships were not well developed, and people were starting to go off sick. No development time had been invested in the team, and eventually the team leader asked for help. The team had a development day with a skilled facilitator, and it transpired that much of the friction within the team was associated with a misunderstanding of roles and confusion over the vision and philosophy of the team.

Care assistants who had previously worked on inpatient wards were working with clients in a way that conflicted with the models of independence that the therapists within the team were trying to promote. For example, a patient had come out of a one-hour session with a physiotherapist where he had to undertake exercises to facilitate independence, but when he went into the communal area, the care assistants did tasks for the individual that the physiotherapist had tried to encourage him to do himself. The care assistants thought they were helping, as this was the work they were familiar and confident with. They did not feel comfortable supervising individuals while they carried out their own tasks, and were much more used to doing these things for people.

Once the team could discuss their philosophy of care and how each team member could contribute to the overall vision and goals of the team, the atmosphere, relationships and quality of care improved significantly.

Economic benefits

We now turn to consider the economic benefits of teamworking. There are two key types of economic benefits that are commonly considered in relation to the impacts of a type of intervention or structure: *cost-effectiveness* (comparing the costs of delivering the same activities and/or specified outcomes between interventions) and *cost-benefits* (total costs in relation to the totality of outcomes). In comparing the costs and benefits of interprofessional teams to other arrangements, studies should (but do not always) include the total costs relating to the organisation and operation of the teams. Examples of such costs are dedicated administrative support time, preparation and attendance of team members at meetings, and related travel expenses.

Lemieux-Charles and McGuire (2006) provide mixed evidence of the economic impacts of healthcare teams, with some studies in their review identifying no difference in service usage or cost-effectiveness; where savings were identified, these were balanced by the increased cost of providing care through a team-based approach. More recent work by Ke et al (2013) specifically explored the economic impacts of interprofessional teams in cancer care, heart failure services, palliative care and older people's services. Results were mixed and varied between those indicating that multidisciplinary teams were able to achieve better outcomes at lower costs to those that suggested higher costs but no improved outcomes and every variation in between! In relation to cancer care, the costs of healthcare were between 33 and 50% lower in patients with malignant melanoma, and 20% lower for patients with haematologic malignancies. The latter was due to lower rates of catheter infection, hepatic complications and hyperglycaemia.

Ke et al (2013) conclude that the current evidence does not enable a definitive judgement on the economic benefits to be made. Other studies have not explicitly included economic elements, but the impacts they report could be thought to increase cost-effectiveness and/or cost-benefits. For example, the findings reported above regarding decreased hospitalisation for mental health patients and an increased survival rate for people with cancer may indicate better cost-effectiveness (replacement of expensive hospital services with those in the community) and cost-benefit (people living longer for the same treatment). Box 2.3 has key summary messages.

Box 2.3: Impact of effective teamworking

- Teams can lead to positive impacts for patients and service users, but this depends on teams focusing on better outcomes for those receiving their services and a supportive organisational context.
- Teams can also improve wellbeing and job satisfaction of staff members, and facilitate reflective practice and professional development.
- The economic benefits of teams are yet to be established, although the evidence that they lead to safer services and more preventative models would suggest that there is the potential for improved cost-effectiveness and cost-benefits.

What is the evidence about what enables teamworking?

As highlighted above, much of the research regarding teams focuses on how they work in practice and the factors that contribute to delivering hoped-for improvements. These factors are often described as being in one of two camps – those that positively facilitate, and those that are barriers. In fact, these are often mirror images of the other; for example, a lack of team purpose may be identified as a key barrier in one study, with a clear team purpose an enabler in other. Further, some are reported as being positive in some circumstances and less helpful in a different setting; for example, co-location can enable team members to develop greater awareness and social connections with each other, but can also result in an increasing awareness of difference in values, working conditions and career opportunities! A key issue is the extent to which the expected members actually believe and experience their collective arrangements to be actual teamwork rather than a looser grouping of individuals. This is sometimes denoted by the extent to which teams are 'real' or 'pseudo'.

West and Lyubovnikova (2013, p 26) describe the latter as follows:

> ... a group of people working in an organization who call themselves or are called by others a team; who have differing accounts of team objectives; whose typical tasks require team members to work alone or in separate dyads towards disparate goals; whose team boundaries are highly permeable with individuals being uncertain over who is a team member, and who is not; and/or who, when they meet, may exchange information but without consequent shared efforts towards innovation.

'Pseudo' teams are the mirror image of 'real teams' and are associated with higher levels of errors, accidents and reduced wellbeing (Dawson et al, 2009). In a recent English NHS staff survey, 96% of respondents said that they work in teams, but only 77% said that they had a set of shared objectives, and 79% said they had to communicate closely with each other to achieve these objectives (DH, 2015b). The proportion reporting 'real' teamworking had increased from previous years (where it had been down as low as 50%), which perhaps reflects the emphasis on teams in recent years (Dawson et al, 2009).

A common way of conceptualising the components that will lead to a team being 'real' is that of IPO (input-process-output), in which the required 'inputs' have to interact through a set of 'processes' in order to achieve the desired 'outcomes' (see Figure 2.1). This has been used as the basis of tools and frameworks to support teams in considering their purpose and practice, such as the Aston Team Performance Inventory (see Chapter 4).

In the next section we consider the evidence regarding the workings of interdisciplinary teams in relation to their 'inputs' and 'processes'.

Interdisciplinary team inputs

The size and composition of interdisciplinary teams are perhaps the most debated factors in the literature. A common assumption is that diversity in membership will provide a greater range of professional expertise and experience, enabling a more holistic and nuanced

Figure 2.1: Input-process-output model of team effectiveness

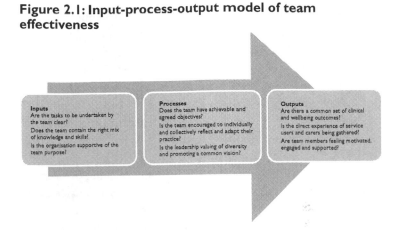

Source: Based on West and Lyubovnikova (2013)

response to service user needs and circumstances. There is evidence to support this with, for example, the study by Borrill et al (2001) finding that greater occupational diversity led to improved effectiveness and more radical innovations. Evans et al (2012) similarly report greater team effectiveness resulting from diversity, providing the example that in mental health teams, social workers may have a different view about the use of compulsory treatment orders than other team members.

The relationship between diversity of members and effectiveness is more complex than thinking that simply increasing one will lead to improvements in the other. Team processes (see below) are vital to ensure that members are positively engaged in the work of the team, and if these do not adapt to increasing diversity, then the potential gains will not be realised (Fay et al, 2006). Also important are different types of membership, which Prades et al (2015) categorise as core, allied and extended. As noted in Chapter 1, the reality is that in some settings individuals will be members of numerous teams during a similar period (O'Leary et al, 2012).

Stability of team membership is also important. In community teams stability is generally related to turnover in staff due to resignation or redeployment to other services, whereas in some surgical procedures it can relate to a handover between professionals in the same operation. Courtenay et al (2013) report that high turnover in the latter setting can lead to a loss of focus and the potential for distraction, which results in longer procedure times. Lyubovnikova and West (2013) extend the notion of diversity beyond professional background, and remind us that gender and ethnicity are also important aspects.

There appear to be numerous issues related to the roles, status and identities connected with different professions. In a general practice setting, for example, these include a lack of clarity between the responsibilities of GPs and practice nurses, GPs seeking to maintain their 'territory' of influence and activity, GPs traditionally being seen as the 'automatic' team leaders, and the inherent hierarchy of one profession owning the business (McInnes et al, 2015). External professions, such as social workers and occupational therapists, also felt perceptions of higher status even though GPs themselves did not always recognise or seek to promote such views (Mangan et al, 2015).

Different professions may also have different perspectives of what good teamwork looks like. For example, nurses in theatre may view this as shared decision-making, whereas doctors describe it as 'having their needs anticipated and directions followed' (Wholey et al, 2014, p 187). This difference may be one reason that studies find doctors rate the standard of teamworking higher than nurses (O'Leary et al, 2012). In relation to dysfunctional teams, Mitchell et al (2014) found the main issue was not the diversity of professions per se, but the extent to which individual professionals identified with their own profession. Strong identification is correlated with increased conflict and less willingness to engage in 'open-minded and elaborative behaviour' (Mitchell et al, 2014, p 7). The topic of professional identification is discussed in more detail in Carpenter and Dickinson (2016).

The physical environment in which the team operates has a bearing on its processes. Sharing the same location, for example, has been shown in some cases to increase familiarity, exchange of information and encourage more open communication in primary and community care settings (Xyrichis and Lowton, 2008). If members are not physically based together, there needs to be other opportunities to interact, through team meetings, online conferencing and other electronic communication options (see Chapter 3).

The broader institutional context that teams are situated in provides another key context. Buttigieg et al (2013) identified three key inputs from organisations regarding team effectiveness: visibility and involvement of management in the life of the team; organisational mission and goals supporting the work of the team; and a management structure that was not overly hierarchical but willing to give teams the autonomy to develop. Weller et al (2011) recommend supportive organisational protocols and procedures as a means to embed good practice in the day-to-day workings of teams. This could range from streamlined paperwork to regular team briefings and opportunities for reflection.

On a similar note, West and Lyubovnikova (2013) highlight research supporting the contribution that care pathways can make in improving communication, relationships and knowledge within teams. Human Resource (HR) systems play a role with individuals who join interdisciplinary teams having to contend with a subsequent lack of career structure, limited opportunities for promotion and a short-term contract or placement connected with time-limited funding (Maslin-Prothero and Bennion, 2010). On a macro level, the legal and policy environments set a broader context. Separate, and at times conflicting, outcome and performance frameworks, financial incentives for uni-disciplinary activity and legal or financial liability sitting with one discipline can all act as barriers (McInnes et al, 2015).

Interdisciplinary team processes

While being clear about overall aims and objectives may seem like the obvious starting point for any initiative, interdisciplinary teams often suffer the same fate as wider integration initiatives in that the purpose and the means to monitor progress are often not established and communicated. A shared vision, particularly when combined with opportunities to frequently interact, help to 'glue' members of a team together through encouraging similar mental models of collaboration and care, and overcoming social boundaries due to professional and organisational differences (Maslin-Prothero and Bennion, 2010). Clear goals and objectives also enable individual team members to be clear about their contribution and how they can best work together (Xyrichis and Lowton, 2008). Performance measurement can help to build a culture of quality improvement (Johnston et al, 2011). West and Lyubovnikova (2013) argue that teams should not only be clear on the objectives, but that these should be of sufficient complexity so that individuals working independently cannot undertake them. Indeed, there is a potential danger of engaging a collective to complete a simple task due to risk of 'social loafing' and 'diffusion of responsibility' (West and Lyubovnikova, 2013, p 137).

Rice (2000) outlines five key assumptions regarding collaborative teamwork. In addition to a shared understanding of roles, values and goals, assumptions also include cooperative working between team members that respects all contributions and a willingness to forgo some autonomy to enable interdependence. Franklin et al (2015) found these to be present in a third to a half of healthcare teams that incorporated community health workers, and suggest that when present, these features enable a shift from traditional hierarchical working to more holistic models of care. Underpinning all of these processes is a need to trust and respect other team members. These are not automatically awarded, and instead have to be earned and developed over time. In primary care settings, GPs have been found to initially not see practice nurses as peers, and to doubt their ability to work autonomously, but with positive experiences they can begin to trust their competence (McInnes et al, 2015).

Courtenay et al (2013) describe the importance of individual members having 'valued commodities' that they can use as the basis of exchange with their peers. These include technical skills and knowledge, access to equipment and resources, and mastery of a clinical territory. Team members commonly cite communication as a means to resolve interdisciplinary conflict along with ensuring that members feel engaged with the work of colleagues (Xyrichis and Lowton, 2008). Group forums are an obvious means for promoting communication, with Prades et al (2015) defining three forms of such forums within cancer care: meetings (discussions of selected patients by professionals); clinics (in which patients are simultaneously examined by team members); and online conferences (used to enable discussion between professionals in geographically spread locations). Interprofessional education is one means to support team members as individuals and as a group to develop the values, skills and knowledge to collaborate successfully (Lyubovnikova and West, 2013). One option is for teams to train together, and this has been reported to prevent errors and improve patient safety in surgery (Weller et al, 2011). Simulations are one option for such training, with one meta-analysis highlighting large effects on clinician behaviours and moderate effects on patient care (Cook et al, 2011). Another book in this series, by Carpenter and Dickinson (2016), explores the topic of interprofessional education in more detail.

A designated coordinator can facilitate the smooth functioning of interdisciplinary teams (Xyrichis and Lowton, 2008; Prades et al, 2015). Such a role helps to ensure that key practicalities and processes are coordinated – this includes those related to the *internal* working of the team, and its interaction with the *external* organisation and other teams (Prades et al, 2015). Coordination also often plays an important role in the leadership of the team, a commonly found key factor in their success or otherwise (Xyrichis and Lowton, 2008). Sakran et al (2012), for example, report a positive relationship between team efficiency and the perception of leadership by team members. Positive leaders used supportive behaviour and constructive feedback to encourage and motivate, and a willingness to adopt collaborative rather than uni-disciplinary and authoritarian decision-making enhanced overall team performance (Courtenay et al, 2013). Despite the importance of leadership, West and Lyubovnikova (2013) report that only 1 in 10 mental health teams and 1 in 3 primary care teams describe having a clear leader.

Another book in this series, by Dickinson and Carey (2016), discusses leadership in more detail, but the key messages from this literature are that there is no one model of leadership or one way to do this effectively that works across the board. Thinking about the adaptive nature of leadership is an important task, which means ensuring that people are clear about the purpose of the team and leadership exercise, the skills and abilities of those they lead, and that they pay attention to factors such as culture and behaviour.

An emerging aspect of interdisciplinary team processes is engagement of service users. This reflects a general recognition that people in receipt of services have a fundamental right to be involved in decisions over their care and treatment, and that effective intervention often relies on their active participation and adoption of new behaviours. Despite increasing emphasis on interprofessional collaboration and service user engagement, these are often developed as parallel, rather than interconnected, initiatives (Martin and Finn, 2011). However, there are a few studies that buck this more general trend. Bilodeau et al (2014) explored patient-centred practice within oncology teams. They found that while patients were welcomed as unique individuals to be treated with respect, teams still tended to make decisions between professionals. This was particularly the case when symptoms did not fit the usual pattern of that condition. Linked to this, while professionals talked about the importance of patient-centred practice, many continued with professionally orientated behaviours, and these were seen to be encouraged by organisational priorities.

Successful pilots in Martin and Finn's (2011) study of projects in NHS cancer-genetic services were able to incorporate service users as 'insiders' within teams. This was achieved through the recruitment of individuals who were seen to have the right motivations and skills, and frequent physical meetings that engaged all team members. It also appeared that professionals and service users were keen to develop informal bonds, and that in some cases they were closer than the professional members within other teams. Direct involvement of service users has also been shown to be a key element for effective interprofessional training (see Carpenter and Dickinson, 2016, this series, for further exploration).

Box 2.4 summarises the key points covered in this section in terms of the enablers of interdisciplinary teamworking. We return to many of these issues in the remainder of the book, setting out case studies of how organisations have dealt with these issues, and frameworks that you may wish to use in your own organisational context.

Box 2.4: Enablers of teamworking

- Diversity within a team provides greater experience and skills that can result in more holistic and creative responses to the needs of patients and service users. But this is only true if the 'right' team processes are in place.
- Perceived differences in status and power between team members can prevent the positive benefits of interdisciplinary teams being realised.
- Leadership and coordination are essential for communication and cooperation within a team, and in developing positive relationships with external teams.
- Clear objectives are essential to provide a vision of what success will look like, and for team members to understand their individual contribution.
- Service users are not commonly engaged in teamworking, but where this has been achieved, there are benefits for all concerned.
- The physical, technological, organisational and policy context in which a team operates have an influence on its internal processes.

Reflective exercises

1. Reflect on your own professional identity – what has shaped this, and how does it affect your interactions with those from different backgrounds?
2. How do the teams that you work in or lead keep service users and carers at the heart of their purpose and decisions? Could this be strengthened?
3. Identify a team that you enjoyed working in, and one that was less positive. What factors contributed to these differing experiences?
4. What evidence does your team gather to understand its impact? Does this look at mainly process and resources, and if so, how could it also consider service user outcomes?
5. Is there a commitment within your organisation to support teamwork? Is this based on recognition of what makes a 'real' team, or could it lead to 'pseudo' teamworking being encouraged?

Further reading and resources

Good places to go regarding evidence of teamworking in health and social care are as follows:

- The Health Services Management Centre (HSMC) at the University of Birmingham. This is one of the leading centres in the UK for the provision of research, teaching, professional development and consultancy to health and social care agencies. For more than 40 years, it has been conducting high-quality, original, policy-relevant research into the organisation, coordination and effectiveness of health and social care service, and helps to shape policy and practice in the UK and abroad: www.birmingham.ac.uk/schools/social-policy/ departments/health-services-management-centre/index.aspx
- The Institute for Research and Innovation in Social Services (Iriss) is a charitable company working to enhance the capacity and capability of the social services workforce in Scotland by enabling access to, and promoting the use of, knowledge and research for service innovation and improvement: www.iriss.org.uk
- *Health and Social Care in the Community,* an international peer-reviewed journal with a multidisciplinary audience: http://onlinelibrary.wiley. com/journal/10.1111/%28ISSN%291365-2524
- The *Journal of Integrated Care* is the UK's leading journal looking at practice, policy and the research of integrated care: www. emeraldinsight.com/journal/jica
- The *Journal of Interprofessional Care* aims to disseminate research and new developments in the field of interprofessional education and practice: www.tandfonline.com/action/ journalInformation?show=aimsScope&journalCode=ijic20#. VioDGH7nvlU
- The International Foundation for Integrated Care is an international collaboration that hosts the *International Journal of Integrated Care* (IJIC), an open-access journal: www.integratedcarefoundation.org/ and http://integratedcarefoundation.org/ijic-international-journal-integrated-care

3

Hot topics and emerging issues

As suggested earlier, teamworking is a diverse field, and the potential literature that may be drawn on is significant and increasing in both breadth and depth. Space means that we cannot talk in detail about all areas that may be important in the future, such as geographically dispersed teams, self-managed teams and team coaching. Changes in the ways we commission and provide services is creating teams that are geographically dispersed away from the main organisational hub, not just across local borders, but in other parts of the country. This provides a range of challenges regarding the support for these teams and their alignment with the host organisation. Self-managed teams come in and out of fashion, but cuts to management layers, a greater understanding of how people engage with services, the need for people to take responsibility for their actions, and decisions being made as close to service users as possible, are again driving an interest in self-managed teams. There is much written about coaching as an intervention for individuals. The art of real team coaching is about enabling teams to improve performance, functioning, wellbeing and engagement (Hawkins, 2014), and it is being recognised as an intervention that can have a tangible impact and accelerate the learning and development of a team.

In this chapter we have chosen to concentrate on three key areas that are most salient to health and social care teams, and will likely remain central regardless of the rapidly shifting context in which we find ourselves:

- As the delivery of health and social care becomes more complex, how can organisations and teams recognise and respond to the *emotional needs* and the impact of *emotional labour* in and across teams?
- As improved *quality of care and safety* is becoming an increasingly

recognised tangible outcome of effective teamworking, what do teams, leaders and organisations need to do in order to develop *culture and behaviour* that improves safety for service users and staff?

- As *communication and information transfer* across organisational boundaries continues to be implicated as a major contributor to failures of safety in a number of high-profile cases, how can it be developed to ensure effectiveness in inter-agency settings?

In this chapter we attempt to draw together lessons from a diverse range of areas and fields around these hot topics to supplement our personal experiences and learning. In Chapter 4 we then go on to present a range of frameworks that may be useful to employ – in both theoretical and practical terms – in attempting to form more effective teams.

Emotional needs and emotional labour

As we become more successful in understanding how to treat physical and psychological needs, service users tend to live with a range of co-morbidities. This means that care is increasingly complex, demanding greater attention and skill from individuals and teams, often in circumstances where we don't know the right answers to situations as we haven't seen them before. There is also increasing scrutiny from the press, and social media can communicate negative judgements on staff in an instant. Delivering complex care in such highly pressurised environments can result in significant emotional impact on staff. One way of understanding the response of staff to such pressure is that of 'emotional labour'.

This was first described by Hochschild (1979) as the ability to manage feelings to display publically accepted emotion in work situations. Her work focused on flight attendants, and identified a dissonance where the emotions that people felt often conflicted with what they actually expressed, or were expected to express, in their role. This work has great resonance for teams working in health and social care as there are expectations (and often unwritten rules) around how to portray and manage emotion – from the organisation, the professions, other team members, and individuals themselves. There is an increasing global literature concerning the impact of emotional labour on nursing (see, for example, Cheng et al, 2013; Sawbridge and Hewinson, 2013), but it is pertinent to note that the concept has resonance for everyone involved in delivering health and social care, irrespective of the care setting, seniority or profession. Following a number of high profile inquiries, the question 'how could that happen?' or 'how could they do that?' is often asked. We would argue that key to the response to this question is emotional labour. Sawbridge and Hewinson (2013, p 129) argue that although the emotional cost of caring is recognised in the literature, it is rarely talked about in the media, and the reality is often not appreciated by organisations.

Hawkins (2014, p 35) suggests that the emotional work of the team is a critical dimension to consider for effective teamworking: 'An effective team ... acts as an emotional container that addresses and resolves conflict, aligns the work of all members, provides emotional support across the team, and increases morale and commitment.' Cornwall (2011) argues that organisations are accountable for ensuring the conditions individuals and teams are working in are supportive and conducive to providing quality compassionate care. The example in Box 3.1 illustrates how one NHS board demonstrated such commitment, accountability and support.

Box 3.1: An example of organisational commitment to emotional labour

As part of an ongoing governing body development programme, the board of a clinical commissioning group (CCG) invited their safeguarding team to come to the board development session and present their work, with the aim of:

- exploring and reaffirming the board's collective and individual roles in safeguarding;
- identifying actions around issues, concerns and good practice.

The safeguarding team facilitated an interactive session and helped the board to further understand the growing numbers of referrals to their service, the changing breadth of the work of the team (new safeguarding definitions extend to slavery and radicalisation agendas), roles and responsibilities, and an insight into the serious case reviews they were working with. The team and board then worked together to determine what they needed from each other, so the safeguarding team were supported to enact their role, and the board could be assured.

Clear actions were determined that included developing greater support for the safeguarding team from the board, including therapeutic support, training and career progression, board support in influencing national leadership and a local workforce meeting.

Source: With kind permission of the Sunderland Clinical Commissioning Group

Haigh (2004, p 19) provides a useful framework to consider the emotional needs of staff, presented as qualities of a therapeutic environment where people can flourish in teams. This includes the following:

- *Attachment:* a culture of belonging, in which attention is given to joining and leaving, and staff are encouraged to feel a part of things.

- *Containment:* a culture of safety, in which there is a secure organisational structure and staff feel supported, looked after and cared about within the team.
- *Communication:* a culture of openness, in which difficulties and conflict can be voiced, and staff have a reflective, questioning attitude to the work.
- *Involvement:* a 'living-learning culture', in which team members appreciate each other's contributions and have a sense that their work and perspective is valued.
- *Agency:* a culture of empowerment, in which all members of the team have a say in the running of the place and play a part in decision-making.

On a similar theme, Maben et al (2012) explored the key conditions needed to create quality patient experience, staff satisfaction and engagement. Space to know colleagues, need for control over the job, a supportive local care climate and a positive emotional 'tone' for delivery of care were seen as fundamentally important. Maben et al (2012) also argue for developing a 'family culture' in teams. We would agree with the desire to create a positive emotional tone where people belong, but would argue for a spirit of friendliness. The reality is that not everyone will be 'friends', much as they may not desire to be family. In our experience, a root cause of poor interpersonal relationships and the subsequent impact on team functioning and climate can come from a reluctance to challenge the behaviour and practice of people who are seen as friends.

We explore culture in more depth later in this chapter, but for now it is important to note themes around the human need to belong and to be supported. In the remainder of this discussion on how teams can respond to emotional needs, we consider three core aspects that have been identified: involvement in decision-making, constructive conflict and time and space to think.

Decision-making

Being involved in decision-making is an essential element in people feeling they have some control over their work. There is a large amount of evidence concerning the correlation between people feeling involved in decision-making and their level of engagement in organisations and teams from across all industries (see Macleod and Clarke, 2009). An example that is often cited is the Buurtzorg model of neighbourhood nursing from the Netherlands. Here self-managing teams are empowered, supported and coached to make decisions they have control of. This has had a positive impact on patient outcomes as well as increasing levels of staff motivation and engagement (Gray et al, 2015).

Katzenbach and Smith (1993) argue that 'real' teams are those that are decisive and in control. They accept that this takes time to develop, and assert that there is a delicate balancing act to be undertaken by a team's leader with regards to decision-making. As Øvretveit (1995, p 43) argues, 'the right decisionmaking process is critical for using different professionals' expertise to the best effect and for energy, morale and work satisfaction in teams.' Team decision-making does not mean that everyone has to be involved in every decision. What is crucial is that teams have an agreed process for decision-making, and within that process there is clarity and understanding about when, how and who will (or needs to) be involved.

In our complex world, where expectations are raised and litigation is growing, people can be fearful of making decisions in case they get it wrong or there are unintended consequences. Ballatt and Campling (2011) identify that some life-and-death decisions are based on best probabilities, and often have to be made quickly, under huge pressure. We suggested in Chapter 2 that diversity can have a positive impact, and the example in Box 3.2 demonstrates this in relation to diversity. However, it has also been suggested that there are a maximum number of diverse views above which decision-making becomes too protracted and difficult. Øvretveit (1995, p 42) argues that teams sometimes try to minimise differences. It is perhaps helpful to illuminate his assertions as they are useful in explaining some of the very real issues that have an impact on teamworking, and contribute to the 'emotional climate' in and across teams within health and social care:

- Teams are fearful that differences will be too destructive on team functioning.
- Practitioners have some skills and knowledge in common, which are often seen by professional associations as unique to individual professions, leading practitioners to perhaps fear that national battles could erupt in the team and lead to competition for valued work.
- Some team members wish to defend hard-won autonomy, and fear that if differences in skill and expertise emerge and come to be seen as more important in the team, the consequence could be that one or more professions becomes more dominant, with others losing autonomy.
- Minimising difference is congruent with developing more equal relationships with clients, and therefore equality is encouraged while status symbols and power displays are reduced.

All these seem like legitimate responses when faced by potentially difficult and stressful situations. However, diversity brings different perspectives, experiences and ways of seeing the world, and as such may contribute to passionate and heated debate. Under some circumstances we might encourage this – teams that do not have lively, impassioned debates may be trying too hard to maintain cohesiveness and hence move to a model of 'group think' (Janis, 1972). A substantial proportion of the collaboration literature continually reiterates the importance of harmonious relationships and avoiding undue conflict. However, if team members do not challenge practices or decisions within collaborative settings, they may find that they seriously compromise the quality of their decision-making. Lasley (2005, p 13) warns about the possible missed opportunities in trying to be harmonious, arguing that teams need to understand and learn to work with heightened emotions, as when 'they have tapped into a vein of dynamic energy that feeds conflict, they are connecting with issues that are important to them.'

Box 3.2: The value of diversity in decision-making

Some nursing members of a multidisciplinary community mental health team were struggling to manage their caseload. The effect of this was that they did not have the capacity to take on new referrals, which had an impact on the workloads of other team members, resulting in increasingly strained relationships. Discussion with the wider team showed part of their reluctance to discharge people against the established criteria was a fear of making the wrong decision. And they were struggling to move their practice to a recovery model of care, where service users are supported to be less dependent on services, and should not stay on caseloads indefinitely. It was decided that nursing team members would pair up for supervision with social workers. This worked exceptionally well, as the skills and experiences of the social workers, together with their different ways of 'seeing situations', helped allay fears, and nurses were able to discharge with more confidence.

Constructive conflict

One of the biggest challenges for teamworking is managing conflict, and in particular managing the emotion associated with conflict situations. However, conflict is not necessarily negative (although it is often assumed to be), and may actually have positive impacts on teamworking. Conflict can be defined as occurring where the concerns of two people *appear* to be incompatible. Conflict arises because essentially people see the world differently, and how that difference manifests itself in behaviour can be why conflict has so many negative associations for many people. But if teams are to be effective, they need to find ways of working positively with difference. The Thomas-Kilmann model of conflict handling (Kilmann and Thomas, 1977) is based on a person's behaviour along two basic dimensions:

- *Assertiveness:* the extent to which the individual attempts to satisfy her/his own concerns.
- *Cooperativeness:* the extent to which the individual attempts to satisfy the other person's concerns.

Figure 3.1 describes five specific methods of dealing with conflicts that individuals may adopt:

- *Accommodation:* helps another individual or group achieve their goals, but often at the expense of reaching your own.
- *Collaboration:* works with other individuals or groups to achieve their goals and yours.
- *Compromise:* middle ground where everybody compromises and only achieves some of their goals.
- *Avoidance:* does not reach either their own goals or those of other individuals or groups. Is uncooperative and unassertive.
- *Competition:* pursues own goals at the expense of other individuals or groups reaching their goals.

Figure 3.1: Model of managing conflict

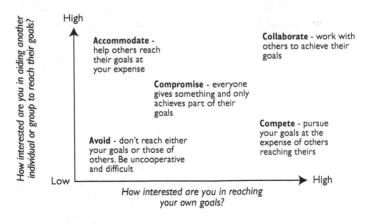

Source: Adapted from Kilmann and Thomas (1977)

The inter-agency working literature typically naturally identifies collaboration as a main objective, but it may be that other styles of working are justifiable dependent on the situation and the task(s) that the specific partnership is faced with achieving. Collaborations may wish to think about where the interests of their agency and those of their partners lie on this matrix, and which models of managing conflict are most appropriate.

Time and space to think

Having argued that being in control of decisions and effectively managing conflict will have a positive impact on teams and climates and relationships, it is important to acknowledge other elements that can contribute to emotional wellbeing. We need leaders and teams to value and believe something that is counterintuitive, that taking time to stop and think to reflect on their work and how they are doing it is fundamental to delivering safe, quality care and wellbeing for patients and staff. Schippers et al (2015, p 769) argue that team reflexivity (the extent to which teams reflect on and adapt their working methods and functioning) is an important predictor of team outcomes, including innovation. What their research also identifies is that team reflexivity has a greater positive impact in teams facing high workloads and demands, even when the physical environment is poor (as it is for so many teams, especially in community settings).

Bridges and Fuller (2014, p 52) identify that team interventions that facilitate workplace learning, empathy, peer support and a positive culture at unit/ward and team level are arguably more effective than development that focuses on individuals. Schwartz Center Rounds are an interdisciplinary initiative from America where groups discuss psychosocial and emotional aspects of care. The one-hour facilitated case-based discussions address a wide range of topics including team conflict and managing mistakes. Research from Lown and Manning (2010, p 1073) identified that participants reported better teamwork, heightened appreciation of role and contributions of others, significant decreases in perceived stress and improved ability to cope with the psychosocial demands of care.

The Schwartz Rounds and situated team reflexivity approach are ways of developing resilience. A common thread of research into resilience is that resilient people and teams are clear about their purpose and access social support to help them to cope (Robertson and Cooper, 2011). Organisations must consider their role in supporting the resilience of their staff and teams. Senior leadership teams, modelling, championing and expecting reflexivity is a very real way of helping teams to become more resilient and to better manage the emotional impact of their work. Box 3.3 sets out the key points to remember about emotional needs and emotional labour.

Box 3.3: Emotional needs and emotional labour

- We need to recognise the emotional cost of caring.
- Well-functioning teams can act as an emotional container for team members.
- People need to be part of decision-making and to feel they have some control over their work.
- We need to help people to work positively with difference.
- Teams need time and space to think and to explore difficult cases and issues.

Culture and safety

Since the first edition of this book, interest in, and understanding of, the importance of teamworking in enhancing safety for patients, service users, carers and staff has grown exponentially. The recognition of culture being fundamental to creating safe environments has been cited in a number of inquiries that span a diverse range of care settings. Dixon-Woods et al (2014, p 106) argue that jurisdictions as far apart as the UK, New Zealand, the Netherlands and the US are experiencing failures in healthcare with similar underlying patterns including cultures of secrecy and protectionism, failing to respond to patient concerns and fragmentation of knowledge. Teamworking (or lack of it) is often a key feature of the inquiries, and we hope that the growing evidence base will persuade people that investment in these processes is really worthwhile.

Within the broader literature one of the factors cited as important in achieving safety is behaviour that creates safe cultures.

Safe cultures

Defining culture is like nailing jelly to a wall – somewhat of a challenge. A frequently used definition is that culture is 'the way we do things around here'. Schein (2004, p 25) argues that we can consider culture at different levels where 'level' means the degree to which cultural phenomena are visible to observers. Schein (2004, p 25) offers three useful levels for us to consider in this chapter.

- *Artefacts:* these include a whole range of things that we can see, hear and feel when we go into a given environment, for example, visible structures, processes, how people communicate and speak to each other, the style of clothes worn, the notices on walls, the stories people tell, if it feels calm or frenetic, how people are welcomed (or not).
- *Espoused values and beliefs:* this second level is about the strategies and goals and rationale for doing things – 'this is how things should be' and why.
- *Underlying assumptions:* this is about the sometimes unconscious beliefs and thoughts driving behaviour and practice in a given environment.

Robert Francis, in his much publicised inquiry into the appalling care at Stafford Hospital (2013, pp 55-6), talked about the dangerous culture that existed at the hospital, where there was:

- lack of openness to criticism
- lack of consideration for patients
- defensiveness
- looking inwards, not outwards
- secrecy
- misplaced assumptions about the judgements and actions of others
- an acceptance of poor standards
- failure to put patients first in everything that was done.

Reflecting the third level in Schein's model, the taken for granted underlying assumption that 'it's just how things are', Francis (2010, p 86) observed that 'There was an acceptance that standards of care, probably through habituation, that should not have been tolerated.' However, what is important to recognise is that not all teams and units in the hospital offered appalling care. The critical question is therefore what was happening in the teams and units that were still able to deliver high quality, innovative care despite the poor organisational culture around them. The answer, unsurprisingly, from all the research we have covered to date, is around leadership, real teamworking and the creation of positive 'safe' cultures within these teams.

Creating 'safe' cultures is not just about creating a team culture that focuses on the issue of safety. It is also about creating a team that has shared commitment to its overall goals and clarity that individuals are accountable not just for their own contribution, but for the quality of the service the whole team delivers. Such a culture means that there is a greater shared interest in services provided, and suggests that individuals have a duty of care to speak up when things are going wrong. The 2013 NHS staff survey (DH, 2015b) showed that only 72% of respondents were confident that it was safe to raise a concern. In response to growing disquiet that some staff were not listened to when they raised concerns and that others were treated poorly when they did, Robert Francis was tasked with undertaking an independent review, which he called *Freedom to speak up*.

> Every organisation involved in providing NHS healthcare should actively foster a culture of safety and learning in which all staff feel safe to raise concerns. (Francis, 2015, p 12)

In situations where there are punitive measures in response to reported incidents or 'near-misses', teams may find that there are much fewer incidents actually reported than in situations where such reports lead to investigations into the real root causes of these events. As Leape (1994, p 1851) identifies, 'ironically, rather than improving safety, punishment makes reducing errors much more difficult by providing strong incentives for people to hide their mistakes, thus preventing recognition, analysis and correction of underlying cause.' Organisations must mean it when they say that they need to learn from errors if learning is to have a positive impact on safety in the future. Quality theorist W. Edwards Deming (quoted in Seddon, 2004) estimates that 95% of the cause of variation in performance is attributable to the system that the work of a team is structured around. In other words, he suggests that failure is due to the way the work is designed and managed, rather than necessarily the people executing the tasks. This might be an overstatement in terms of the importance of structure and process, but most organisational theorists would agree that most significant breakdowns in safety are not purely the result of the actions of an inattentive individual(s), but relate to other systemic influences.

In his book *Life in error* (2013), James Reason introduces a cultural strata framework that builds on earlier typologies developed by Hudson and Westrum. The framework identifies the focus that different organisations take, especially when things go wrong; namely, a systems (learning) approach or a person-centred (blame) approach (see Table 3.1).

Table 3.1: Cultural strata framework

Generative	Respects, anticipates and responds to risks. Strives for resilience and to create a just, learning, flexible, adaptive, prepared and informed culture, where people trust, and there is a real understanding that safety is everyone's business
Proactive	Has an awareness and understanding that that 'latent pathogens' and 'error-traps' are present in the system. Constantly works to eliminate them, and listens to what is happening at all levels of the organisation
Calculative	A culture that dutifully develops and integrates systems to 'manage safety', often in response to external pressures, as it is the right thing to do — a 'by the book' approach
Reactive	A culture where safety is given attention after an event, often driven by concerns about negative publicity. An incident reporting system may be established as something that needs to be in place, but it is a quick fix and does not develop into a system where people can really learn and share learning to help prevent similar situations from happening again
Pathological	Blame, denial and the blinkered pursuit of excellence. Financial targets can dominate with an aim of making things more effective and efficient (cheaper/faster)

Source: Based on Reason (2013)

Psychological safety and trust

The creation of a safe environment is crucial if people are to have the confidence to speak up when things go wrong. Edmondson (2012, p 118) argues that teams need to develop psychological safety, which she defines as 'a climate in which people feel free to express relevant thoughts and feeling.' Psychological safety was sadly missing from some teams and units at the Mid Staffordshire Hospital, and Francis (2013) determined that culture and a lack of individual confidence and skill prevented people speaking up.

It is not only in health and social care where people struggle to give tough messages. The Chartered Institute of Personnel and Development (CIPD) (2013a) identified that the biggest challenge for leaders from across agencies was to manage conflict and have difficult conversations.

Edmondson (2012, p 121) offers four specific perceived personal risks that inhibit an individuals' willingness or ability to speak up: being seen as ignorant, incompetent, negative and disruptive.

Individuals need to feel secure and know that they will not be victimised for speaking up, but developing the confidence to do so means that there must be mutual trust and respect among team members. It is crucial to highlight that trust does not develop easily or quickly; it takes time, and therefore the need for stability in teams arises again. Edmondson's work on medication errors in North American hospitals again adds valuable insight (1996). She identified that leader behaviour was fundamental in developing a climate whereby mistakes and errors could be discussed safely and openly. Teams run in a dictatorial or hierarchical fashion were less likely to report errors than those more horizontally organised with distributed leadership. Additionally, she identified what many others know intuitively, that where there is a climate of trust and openness, reporting of errors may initially rise. It is crucial that team leaders understand these consequences and aim to develop a culture where people are not afraid to share and disclose errors and mistakes. As an example of this, in 2006, figures indicated that the number of racially motivated crimes recorded by the police in England and Wales went up by 12% (Home Office, 2006). However, rather than suggesting that this was negative and indicated an increase in racist incidents, the Association of Chief Police Officers (ACPO) suggested that the rise was in part an indication of the success of work done to encourage victims of such crimes to come forward. In other words, ACPO suggested this rise in reporting illustrated a culture that has become better aware and more sensitive to these kinds of offences.

It is also important to recognise that some teams have two leaders, especially if there are members from different organisations or agencies (or perhaps teams have one leader but report to different managers). A lack of consistency in relation to supporting staff that have made or disclosed errors is divisive, and mitigates against real teamworking. Figure 3.2 illustrates the type of trend we might expect to see in the reporting of near misses when trying to form a more open culture.

Figure 3.2: Expected pattern for near-miss reporting in creating a more open culture

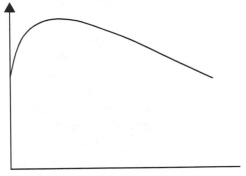

Number of near misses reported

Time

Trust

Curşeu and Schreiber (2010) argue that trust influences team effectiveness directly. The CIPD (2013b) has identified that trust is weaker in the public sector. Although there are high levels of trust between colleagues and line managers, trust in senior managers is much weaker, which can contribute to a 'them and us' mentality. This has significant implications for teamworking. If senior managers don't have positive relationships with teams who are actually delivering services, they are likely to be less well informed or aware of intelligence and tacit knowledge that can have a direct impact on the quality of care delivered.

Boston (2014, p 15), identified seven factors that he argues determine the extent to which others will trust you: an individual's propensity to trust anyone, common ground, your predictability, your proved competence, your integrity, your benevolence and how much you trust them. Reffo and Wark (2014) see things similarly, but also talk about transparency, inclusivity and concern for the best interest of others in their work on politically intelligent leaders. Arguably, to trust someone, you have to have a relationship with them. It is salutary to consider that many of the current ways of working in health and social care mitigate against relationships developing. For example, the high use of temporary agency and bank staff mean it is hard for colleagues, as well as patients, to develop a shared understanding of each other. Additionally, the European Working Time Directive has had a significant impact on how doctors work. Junior doctors have increasingly shorter rotations so aren't able to spend enough time in given areas to develop trust in colleagues (or for trust to develop in them). There is an irony that early on in their careers doctors don't always work as members of well-functioning teams, but end up in senior roles where they are responsible for leading teams (often without the inherent skills or confidence to do so).

Behaviour

There is increasing recognition in organisations that having a set of values is not enough to influence culture. People need to 'live values' if culture is to change, and organisations are increasingly looking to develop a framework of behaviours that are clear, explicit and measurable so that people can understand what is expected of them and their colleagues, and be held to account against these. The impact of 'poor behaviour' cannot be underestimated. Porath and Pearson (2013, p 117) argue that performance and team spirit deteriorated in the organisations they studied as a consequence of rudeness and incivility. Negative consequences include people being less able to focus and colleagues not volunteering to help each other out (Porath and Pearson, 2013). The case study in Box 3.4 highlights a 'board to ward' organisational approach that picks up the power and impact of peer feedback.

Box 3.4: Changing culture and behaviour

The Bethanie Group (Western Australia) is a provider of aged care services and accommodation including residential aged care, community aged care, retirement living and affordable community housing. An internal staff satisfaction survey in 2010 showed that many employees did not enjoy working with their co-workers, and that other working relationships across business levels and between departments were strained. There was a high level of staff turnover and absenteeism, and low cooperation and collaboration.

In February 2011 they appointed a new chief executive officer. His priority and a key performance indicator was to change Bethanie's workplace culture, by changing people's behaviour and mindset. He created a plan linking strategic challenges and business outcomes to changed workplace behaviours, and initiated a series of workshops with employees to identify what it was like to work for Bethanie. This information helped shape the 'Six Signature Behaviours' framework (ultimately called 'Living the Six') that was then successfully implemented across the organisation. Working with organisational psychologists, a 'Culture Pulse' survey, conducted at least three times each year, was developed, which asks all staff to confidentially rate themselves and each member of their team on each of the Six Signature Behaviours.

Culture Pulse is not simply about measuring behaviours. All staff, from the board and executive group through to care staff and operations, have been provided with continuous training on how to positively display Bethanie's Signature Behaviours. An internal Culture Committee has been established and embedded into the governance framework, and there are trained culture change advocates at each site. The executive group and the board are committed and involved. All staff receive formal training focusing on how to translate the Signature Behaviours into day-to-day work, and every new employee is introduced to the Signature Behaviours on the first day of employment at their staff induction programme.

Since the introduction of Culture Pulse to the organisation in May 2011, multiple key performance indicators have improved. Staff engagement has increased, retention rates have gone from 58% to 75%, absenteeism has declined, and the use of (outside) agency staff to cover shifts has also declined and profitability has increased.

Source: Example provided by Steve Becsi (Global CEO, Pulse Australasia), with thanks also to McDonald (2014)

Learning

Culture, safety and trust are all critical if teams are to deliver quality care, but the Department of Health in England correctly asserts that a 'culture that is honest, that listens and that finds and faces the truth is not enough. It must be accompanied by learning, and by change for the better' (DH, 2015a, p 10). Buchanan (2011) reflects on why we don't learn, and cites the examples of Victoria Climbié and Peter Connolly, both children who died after suffering appalling abuse. Their deaths were separated by seven years, and the Public Inquiry chaired by Lord Laming (2003) after Victoria's death blamed a catastrophic systematic failure among the agencies responsible for safeguarding vulnerable children. So the question is, why didn't we learn from Victoria's death and adapt practice? Buchanan distinguishes between extreme and routine contexts, and suggests that changes following extreme contexts often have defensive agendas, which are focused on preventing things from happening and managing risks, together with often-inflammatory media commentary, externally imposed agendas and a lack of good change agent support. He further argues that we can't assume (as we seem to) that receptivity to change will be high in these circumstances or that it will be easy (Buchanan, 2011, p 273).

A learning culture is one where people are interested in understanding what has happened, why it happened and then take steps to ensure that it doesn't happen again. Moreover, learning organisations share their learning and experiences widely in order to prevent errors and enhance safety. Health and social care agencies are starting to do this, but have a long way to go to catch up with airlines that have an advanced system for sharing lessons across diverse and often competing organisations (see, for example, Hamman, 2004). Edmondson (2012) talks about work in groups needing collective learning, and identifies that individuals need to contribute by asking questions, sharing information, seeking help, talking about mistakes, seeking feedback and trying new things out.

The key summary points relating to culture changes are set out in Box 3.5.

Box 3.5: Culture changes

- Culture and climate have an impact on staff and patient wellbeing and safety.
- People need to feel psychologically safe if they are to raise issues about things that are going wrong.
- People need to find ways to develop trust in each other.
- Behaviour matters – organisations and teams must find ways of being clear about acceptable behaviour.
- Creating a real learning culture is essential if teams are to be innovative and safe.

Communication and information transfer

We communicate all the time. Indeed, it is imperative for our very survival on a day-to-day basis. Yet communication is at the heart of many of the issues that have risen to prominence in relation to poor practice in health and social care that have often had negative consequences for patients. Dunn et al (2007, p 213) highlight that this is a global issue, arguing that communication failure was involved in approximately 75% of more than 7,000 cause analysis reports to the Department of Veterans Affairs' National Center for Patient Safety in the US. In the UK, the evidence from the Health and Social Care Information Service (2014) is clear: written and oral communication, along with the attitude of staff (how messages are delivered), forms the second highest number of complaints against health and social care services.

There are a range of issues that influence the sending and receiving of messages in everyday situations. Sutcliffe et al (2004, p 186) argued that in addition to poor information exchange, communication is a complex concept associated with hierarchical differences, the ability to influence upwards, conflicting roles, role ambiguity, interpersonal power and conflict. Many of the points we make in this section are relatively straightforward or intuitive, but in the fast-paced environment of service delivery, elements of best practice can become overlooked. One such point is that we cannot assume how others will interpret and act on (or whether they have the facilities to act on) any communications we make. A quote from the Victoria Climbié Inquiry illustrates this starkly: 'I cannot account for the way other people interpreted what I said. It was not the way I would have liked it to have been interpreted' (Laming, 2003, p 9). Although communication is often taken for granted as something we do all the time, effective communication is much more difficult to achieve in practice, and involves not only the sending of a message, but its receipt and interpretation. Although we may think that we have said (or written) something that is relatively straightforward or comprehensible, there are a number of factors that influence whether this is the case, such as personal style, communication technologies, professional discourse and language.

Communicating with service users

Much of what is written about communication in health and social care is concerned with the ways in which professionals, agencies and organisations interact. However, this often misses a key element of the jigsaw – the service user. In terms of written messages it is suggested that more attention needs to be paid to the literacy level of service users, and that we should not assume that everyone has the same reading ability. If we define effective teamworking as meeting the needs of service users, it is sobering to reflect the extent of societal challenge in the UK with regards to literacy. For example, teams working with offenders – often across very complicated pathways and boundaries – need to consider that 48% of prisoners have literacy skills at or below Level 1 and 65% have numeracy skills at or below Level 1 (Natale, 2010). More than one-third of people in prison have a reading level below Level 1 and 75% below Level 1 for writing (Level 1 is generally accepted as what we might expect of an 11-year-old).

A study aiming to improve communication between Aboriginal patients and healthcare workers in Australia (Cass et al, 2002) reached conclusions that are pertinent for everyone delivering care to consider, namely, that miscommunication is pervasive. We often don't recognise it is happening, and factors include lack of control by the patient, differing modes of discourse, a dominance of the medical model, a lack of shared understanding and knowledge, cultural and linguistic differences and a lack of training for staff in intercultural communication, together with failure to access professional interpreters.

The world is turbulent and changing quickly, with many countries now challenged to meet the health and social care needs of migrants. A study by Butow et al (2011, p 285) into migrant perceptions of communication with a cancer team identified that some patients felt they were 'in a bubble', able to see, but unable to communicate with the outside world. This prevented them from expressing their needs and concerns, inhibiting them from receiving the reassurance and support they needed.

It is not just the spoken word that needs attention, however. The Health Service Ombudsmen (cited in *British Medical Journal*, 2004, p 10) lamented, 'if only all health service staff made sure they listened to patients and their carers, communicated clearly with them and with each other, then made a note of what had been said, the scope for later misunderstanding and dispute would be reduced enormously.'

Personal style and non-verbal communication

Individual communication style is important, as we are all different. In this book we argue that if teams are able to capitalise on the differences of their members, then they have the potential to be more effective. To do this, however, we need to invest time in exploring and understanding differences to harness these positively. In terms of spoken communication, one such factor is non-verbal communication (that is, body language). Mehrabian (1972) suggests that this forms 70% of the message, whereas the words themselves are only 7% of the message, and the tone of the delivery carries 23% of the message. This is well worth reflecting on and thinking about just how well we really know our communication abilities. Individuals often have somewhat of a blind spot in relation to their ability to communicate effectively, and it is a useful exercise to think about how others might see and hear us. Personal preferences and style have an impact on communication, and it is helpful for team members to consider their style and how they may misunderstand the intent and actions of others. The Myers Briggs Type Indicator is one of many psychometric tools that aim to create personal and interpersonal awareness. It focuses on preference across four dimensions, and each has an impact on how we communicate and work with others (see, for example, Briggs Myers and Myers, 1995; Briggs Myers, revised by Kirby and Myers, 2000):

- *Energy source:* people with a preference for *extraversion* get energised by doing things and being with others (they prefer to talk things through) while people with a preference for *introversion* get their energy from an internal world of memories, thinking and reflection (they think things through).
- *Type of information:* people with a preference for *sensing* prefer facts and focus their attention on detail, practicality and what is happening in the present. Those with a preference for *intuition* are interested in connections, associations, the big picture and future possibilities.
- *How decisions are made: thinking* is about taking decisions in an analytical, logical, objective way, removed from the situation. *Feeling* is concerned with making decisions based on values around people, and tries to empathise and understand from a people perspective.
- *Preference for living life: judging* is a preference for living in a structured, organised, planned way, often driven by deadlines, and *perceiving* is a preference for living in a more flexible way that keeps options open until the last minute.

We view the world from our own lens, and if you consider that we often appoint people in teams in our likeness (unconscious bias), we can see how some people's needs can go unrecognised or may be misconstrued.

Communication technologies and information transfer

We all form snap judgements about people as they do about us, and we need to reflect on how this can have an impact on our communication with others. Working across multiple sites may not necessarily have a negative impact on communication between members given the rise of different communication technologies, as research into virtual teams is demonstrating. Virtual teams offer increased flexibility, reduced travel time and expense, access to the best resources regardless of location, and 24-hour workdays on projects. Research into virtual teams demonstrates that we need to pay attention to language and style (virtual etiquette), as well as to cultural dimensions if we are to effectively communicate and collaborate on projects (Lee, 2014). In reality, access to, confidence and support to use technologies varies enormously. As such, we need to pay close attention to the modes of communication that we use, and where and when these forms are and are not more suitable in comparison with others.

Unlike the vast majority of acute services, not all staff members working in the community can easily access computer and printer facilities. There are undoubtedly major systemic issues that need investing in if teamworking is to be as effective as possible, and these do not always mean spending large amounts of money. Often firewalls limit the size of information that can be sent, or organisations may restrict use of video communication tools such as Skype or Zoom (as there are concerns about breaches of safety and confidentiality). Investing small sums and empowering teams to be able to spend wisely can make a real difference. A number of evaluations of inter-agency working have cited IT as a major barrier to information sharing (Richardson and Asthana, 2005). A Department of Health report found that the information aspects of collaborative working lag well behind (Rhodes, 2003).

Problems may include legal information-sharing barriers, difficulties with incompatible IT systems or a lack of common referral systems (Cameron and Lart, 2003). However, simply improving information systems or using them more extensively will not necessarily produce more effective communication or teamwork. Although it is clearly important that professionals are able to communicate well, and IT aids this to an extent (particularly when teams are not co-located), it is a myth that by simply getting this right teams will be able to function effectively, just as it is a myth that by structuring organisations/teams in the 'right' way they will automatically be more successful.

There is a significant amount written in the literature about using handovers and checklists to support safe communication, taking away dependence on fallible human memory (see Chapter 4 for frameworks and tools). But handovers don't always contribute to effective communication and the delivery of safe care, as the following example from research into a large intensive care unit illustrates:

> A huge amount of time is spent in handover and rounds – with some rounds taking 3 hours. The rounds observed raise questions about people's attention spans and concentration during such long periods and many discussions were interrupted or people had to leave the round. A walk around medical handover appeared to be constantly interrupted and senior nursing staff were struggling to fully understand the decisions and actions needed. Sometimes the handover structure appears to cause delay in nurses implementing treatment changes. For example, on one occasion, issues and changes to treatments discussed at the 8am handover had still not been amended on the treatment chart by the time the formal ward round visited the patient at 12.30pm. (Jelphs, 2008)

Conversely, the example in Box 3.6 illustrates how a handover tool can contribute to more effective communication within a team.

Box 3.6: Handover in a specialist mental health team

Team dynamics in a well-respected interprofessional mental health team were fraught. The consultant felt that everyone deferred to him to make decisions, and that other team members weren't taking responsibility or using their knowledge and expertise effectively. Team coaching with the three senior leads identified that there was no agreed way to share information, and a lot of assumptions were being made. The consultant was getting stressed and people were reluctant to approach him, creating a vicious cycle where communication around this high-risk group was compromised. Introducing a specific structured handover tool (see Chapter 4) has made a real difference to the quality of information shared, interprofessional relationships and the team climate.

Nagpal et al (2012) researched care across a whole surgical pathway, finding lack of communication between teams. Even where information was available it was fragmented and difficult to access, compromising patient safety. Lingard (2012, p 20) argues for more research around intertextuality to help us understand how communication (or lack of it) at one stage of care ('upstream') can shape, often invisibly, patient safety events at a later stage. She argues that meaning and understanding can get lost and distorted as people move from oral and written communication, and this can have a major impact at transition points between care settings and agencies. The Hurricane Katrina example (see Box 1.1 in Chapter 1) showed how poor communication contributed to catastrophic damage. Research into the aftermath of Hurricane Katrina showed a level of 'disinformation' – even when information was being sent by email to hand-held devices, individuals purported not to have received this, disconnecting decision-makers and those with power from the responders on the ground (Piper and Ramos, 2006). Studies analysing the use of IT in child safeguarding (Dickinson, 2014) identify similar concerns about the ways that professionals work across boundaries and how information is shared (or not). The example in Box 3.7 demonstrates how one organisation is working to share information across boundaries and support practitioners.

Box 3.7: Patchwork and information sharing

Patchwork operates in the UK and Australia with the aim of connecting care workers across agencies around shared clients. The system allows the sharing of basic information without compromising sensitive case management data and the raising of concerns around individual clients. They identify that care workers spend a significant amount of time trying to contact people at other agencies – with more than half spending somewhere between one and six hours weekly trying to track their colleagues down.

They argue that when care workers understand the full picture of how their clients interact with public services, it's much easier for them to coordinate their efforts before situations escalate and interventions are required. At the time of writing 1,894 professionals across the UK and Australia are currently supporting 5,375 clients through Patchwork, enabling a higher quality of care, safeguarding of vulnerable clients and increased productivity for front-line staff.

> 'When I see a child with bruises, I have a 10 minute appointment slot to decide whether I need to raise a concern. With Patchwork, I have instant access to colleagues that can help me make a better decision for the child.' (GP, Staffordshire)

Source: See http://patchworkhq.com

Professional discourse and language

The sociological field of research describes professions as self-interested groupings where professionals are socialised into groups that hold a particular professional identity that can become a valued part of an individual's personal identity (Evetts, 1999). The process of professional training not only passes on 'official' learning in the sense of the technical skills with which professionals are imbued, but also serves to institutionalise professionals into certain ways of acting and thinking. That is, individuals become part of a particular professional discourse that provides a social boundary that defines what can be said about a specific topic, or what might be considered the limits of acceptable speech (for a practical example of this within mental health services, see 6 et al, 2007). Discourse has an impact not only on what it is possible to say, but also on the ways in which communications are made.

By understanding that professionals think and communicate in different ways and find different forms of information acceptable, individuals may find that they react differently to communication with other professions. Rather than reacting in an aggressive way, they may have a better comprehension of why professionals communicate in particular ways and try to overcome these, rather than dismissing information that does not fit their particular discourse. Sheehan et al (2007) argue that there are distinct differences in the sophistication of communication between multidisciplinary and interprofessional teams. Their research identified that multidisciplinary team members worked and communicated in parallel ways, not really sharing or considering the wider significance of specific information. Interprofessional teams demonstrated a more inclusive language, were more collaborative and continually shared information. Interprofessional teams tried to create their own language, one that was acceptable and understood by the different professions. Hayes (2011) believes that the language teams develop reflects and reinforces their prevalent culture. By creating an opportunity for teams to become aware of the language they use, this can help them learn, develop, and arguably form better relationships with other teams. Box 3.8 reiterates the key points regarding communication.

Box 3.8: Communication

- Poor communication is a major contributor of poor quality care and serious incidents.
- We need to challenge ourselves around the quality of communication with service users.
- Understanding our personal communication styles will mean we can communicate more effectively with others who are different.
- Information does not transfer easily and clearly across boundaries.
- Structured handover tools used well can help the quality of information being shared.
- Technology can help – if we learn how to use it well and appropriately.

This chapter has highlighted the complexity and interdependency of the inputs, systems and processes needed for effective teamworking, and we have outlined some frameworks that may aid professionals in navigating these.

The next chapter outlines more practical tools that will be useful for teams operating in inter-agency settings.

Reflective exercises

In response to these questions, think about a team you are a member of. If you are not currently a member of a team, think of a time in the past when you have been a member of a work team, or else, think of a team that you have been a member of in your personal life or a team you have read about.

1. How often does your team meet, or spend quality reflexive time together?
2. Reflect on the therapeutic framework considering the emotional needs of teams – does your team have these conditions in place?
3. Consider the cultural strata framework (Table 3.1) illustrated in this chapter. Which level reflects practice in your team?
4. Reflect on an adverse incident that has taken place in a team you have experience of. What did you think, what did you feel, and what did you do in this situation?
5. How would you describe the language used in your team – is it accessible to everyone?
6. Take time to consider communication in your 'home' team (the work team you spend most time with). What image or metaphor would you use to describe the reality of communication? What does this tell you about communication in your team, and with other teams? And what improvements would you like to see?

Further reading and resources

This chapter has covered a broad range of issues, and readers may want to follow up specific topics in more detail. The further reading and resources below are diverse to enable individuals to explore all the issues that are relevant to them and their local context.

- For further exploration of communication issues see Stanton's (2003) *Mastering communication*.

- The Social Care Institute for Excellence report by Bostock et al (2005), *Managing risk and minimising mistakes to services for children and families*, may be a useful resource in aiding professionals to think through how they could better report near-misses and produce organisational learning that avoids major incidents.

- This video session delivered at the University of Birmingham by Yvonne Sawbridge for TEDx asks the question 'Why might good people deliver bad care?': www.youtube.com/watch?v=VC4FajTFpRUU

- For research information and free tools around measuring resilience, see: www.robertsoncooper.com/iresilience/

- For information on global trends on trust, access the 2015 Edelman Trust Barometer: www.edelman.com/2015-edelman-trust-barometer/

- For information on Schwartz Centre Rounds, see: www.theschwartzcenter.org/

- For more insight into personal preferences and styles (including Myers Briggs), access the OPP website at: www.opp.com/en/tools/MBTI/MBTI-Step-I

- NHS Improving Quality (NHS IQ) is the driving force for improvement across the NHS in England, working to improve health outcomes for people by providing improvement and change expertise: www.nhsiq.nhs.uk/

- The Department for Business, Innovation and Skills has a range of tools and literature on employee engagement: www.gov.uk/government/organisations/department-for-business-innovation-skills

4

Useful frameworks and concepts

Throughout this book we have tried to convey the message that just concentrating on supporting individual teams is not enough in the complex world of health and social care delivery. It's a bit like baking a cake – you may have the very best quality ingredients, but it is how they interact together that is the predicator of a cake that is well baked and delicious to eat. Historically, significant effort has gone into developing single teams, while not perhaps recognising or paying enough attention to the environment that teams operate within. In this revised edition we also focus on the individual's responsibility for being a team member. How we show up as individuals and contribute (or not) on a day-to-day basis has an impact on both the culture (how we do things around here) and climate (how it feels) of the team and its relationships with other teams.

This chapter is structured around four interdependent levels that need to work together if teams are to ultimately succeed: individual, team, organisation and partnership. We introduce a range of models, frameworks and tools that have been successfully tried and tested in teamworking in and across a variety of organisational settings. It was difficult to choose which models and frameworks to include as there are literally hundreds (this has involved robust debate and negotiation, as in all the best teams!). Models and frameworks are sometimes perceived as only having academic relevance, but they are a way of representing the reality of the world, and can help in making sense of what sometimes seem overwhelmingly complex situations and issues (while acknowledging that models are not inevitably direct reflections of the world we live in).

For each model and framework introduced we briefly explore what they are trying to do, when they could be used, and provide suggestions for use in practice. The further reading and resources section at the end of this chapter has been designed to signpost readers to a wider range of tools to complement this material, and also highlights ideas that we were not able to explore in detail here.

Tools and frameworks for individuals

Personal contribution: What is expected?

We don't all like working in teams. The reality is that for many people it is not a preference, but the complexity of care today (and professional codes of conduct) demand positive interaction with and between teams. A useful, but perhaps uncomfortable thing to do, is to reflect on our personal contribution and ways of working.

What does it seek to explore?

The 'What is expected?' personal reflective exercise in Box 4.1 seeks to enable individuals to reflect on their personal contribution to the teams they are working in. The framework captures some of the ways in which team members need to contribute, highlights expectations that others have of us, and may serve to challenge our thinking.

When to use it

This reflective exercise could be used in a variety of ways. For example, if individuals are frustrated by how the team is working, they may like to reflect on their own contribution. They may have had feedback about their personal contribution that they don't think is fair or balanced. The framework could be used in preparation for an appraisal, supervision or coaching session. Additionally, people who are working in and across a number of teams (which is the reality for many) may like to reflect on their different contributions in different settings.

Suggestions for use in practice

Take time to reflect on the questions posed in Box 4.1. Try to answer honestly (not what you would perhaps like the answers to be), and explore why you may be contributing in certain ways. Remember that motivation and intent are different to behaviour – what people are seeing and experiencing may not be what you are intending them to see and feel.

Alternatively, work through the questions with a trusted colleague, and ask them to give honest feedback, in order to help you further understand your contribution to the team you are working in.

Box 4.1: What is expected?

- Do you attend team meetings, and how do you contribute?
- Do you take part in reviewing how the team is working to achieve its objectives?
- Do you work to deliver the team objectives?
- Are you committed to the purpose of the team and other team members?
- How do you question and challenge – is it constructive or consistently negative?
- Do you participate in decision-making?
- Do you share information?
- Do you take time to listen?
- Do you share your knowledge, skills and learning?
- Do you help to create a culture of trust, support and safety?
- How do you talk about the work of the team with other teams and stakeholders?

Individual team roles: Belbin team role descriptions

The work of Meredith Belbin and colleagues at Henley Management College in the 1970s set out to explore why some teams work and others don't. Over time, their research with international management teams revealed that the difference between success and failure for individual teams was not dependent on intellectual ability (IQ), but on how people behaved. The research identified groups of behaviours that form distinct ways in which people contribute to teams, known as team roles. There are now nine identified team roles. In addition to the appointed functional roles of individuals it is suggested that effective teams have people with a number of different roles, and really effective teams comprise people from across the spectrum of roles (again, highlighting the importance of diversity).

What does it seek to explore?

The Belbin team role descriptions enable individuals and teams to explore their preferred team behaviour or 'team role'. Roles don't always stay static, and it is not unusual for people to identify with more than one. The nine roles, with their contribution and allowable weaknesses (the flipside to the strength of the role, which is allowable because of the strengths the roles brings), are detailed below, in Table 4.1.

When to use it

Understanding your team roles is helpful for both individuals and teams. Working in areas of strength and preference can help with motivation and feeling understood and belonging.

Suggestions for use in practice

This can be helpful in illuminating differences and preferences, and help teams understand each other better. Teams could use this when newly formed, seeking to understand each other and to work out how they could best use each other's skills and preferences. Alternatively, this is useful for teams to use when they have been together for a while and are considering how to further develop, or are struggling to work together well.

Table 4.1: Belbin team role descriptions

Team role	Contribution	Allowable weaknesses
Plant	Creative, imaginative, free-thinking; generates ideas and solves difficult problems	Ignores incidentals; too preoccupied to communicate effectively
Resource investigator	Outgoing, enthusiastic, communicative; explores opportunities and develops contacts	Over-optimistic; loses interest once initial enthusiasm has passed
Coordinator	Mature, confident, identifies talent; clarifies goals; delegates effectively	Can be seen as manipulative; offloads own share of the work
Shaper	Challenging, dynamic, thrives on pressure; has the drive and courage to overcome obstacles	Prone to provocation; offends people's feelings
Monitor evaluator	Sober, strategic and discerning; sees all options and judges accurately	Lacks drive and ability to inspire others; can be overly critical
Teamworker	Cooperative, perceptive and diplomatic; listens and averts friction	Indecisive in crunch situations; avoids confrontation
Implementer	Practical, reliable, efficient; turns ideas into actions and organises work that needs to be done	Somewhat inflexible; slow to respond to new possibilities
Completer finisher	Painstaking, conscientious, anxious; searches out errors; polishes and perfects	Inclined to worry unduly; reluctant to delegate
Specialist	Single-minded, self-starting, dedicated; provides knowledge and skills in rare supply	Contributes only on a narrow front; dwells on technicalities

Source: Reproduced by kind permission of Belbin®

Trust: Boston's model of trust

Throughout this book there has been a theme of the importance of individuals and teams having trust in each other. The Edelman Trust Barometer argues that trust in senior leaders and institutions is decreasing globally. Research consistently tells us that trust in individual line managers is critical for staff to feel engaged. In his book, *ARC leadership* (where ARC = authentic, responsible, courageous), Richard Boston (2014) introduces a model of trust that is helpful as a reflective tool for individuals and teams (see Figure 4.1).

What does it seek to explore?

The model is made up of seven factors that Boston argues determine the extent to which someone will trust you, whatever your relationship with them. Let's just consider a few elements of the model:

- *Common ground:* in teams, the common ground that connects people, whatever their profession, discipline or expertise, is the drive to contributing to safe effective quality care. Reminding ourselves of common ground that is often lost in the challenges of day-to-day working and competing pressures is really important.
- *Predictability:* predictability and behaving consistently help people know how we are going to react, which is important if we are to earn other's trust (although Boston makes the important point that effective leaders need to be flexible in their behaviour to match given situations and the individual need of their followers, which is a paradox to consistency).
- *Personal integrity:* we can all be critical of others, but do we always act with the integrity we demand of others?

When to use it

This model provides us with a way of exploring a concept that can, at times, seem intangible. Individuals can use this tool to critically reflect on their behaviour and contribution in individual and team settings. Teams can use this tool when considering their relationship with other teams. Mature teams could consider some or all of the elements and relationships within the team itself.

Suggestions for use in practice

The model can be printed out (whole, or as individual elements), screened as a PowerPoint slide or written on a flipchart. The team can take individual elements, exploring each in turn, before considering if this requires action.

Figure 4.1: Model of trust

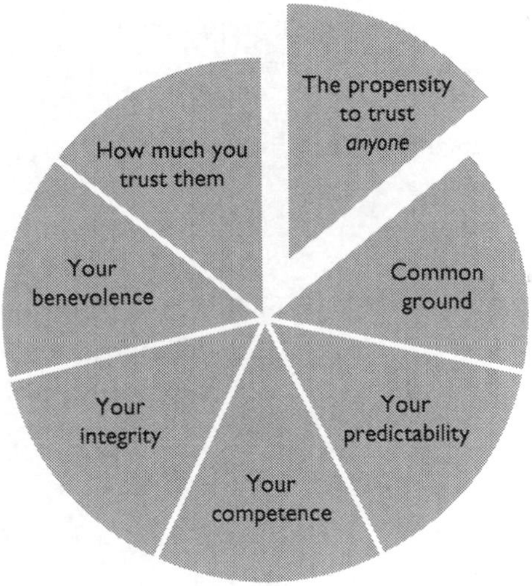

Source: Boston (2014)

Tools and frameworks for teams

Ideas in this section can be used by individual teams or used flexibly to consider teamworking across boundaries. We start by considering the important issue of role clarity.

Role of members: Role clarity review grid

The importance of role clarity cannot be underestimated. Examples in this book have shown that confusion over roles can lead to poor relationships, stress, a negative impact on service users and possible duplication of work. The Belbin model introduced earlier explored what behavioural roles people may adopt in teams (see Table 4.1). The role clarity review grid introduced here focuses on functional and professional roles in teams (see Table 4.2).

What does it seek to explore?

Effective interprofessional teamworking is about producing synergy, where the combined effect of all professional contributions exceeds the sum of the potential individual effects. Synergy may come from:

- *understanding* roles, skills, knowledge, expertise, ambitions
- *respecting* beliefs, working style
- *valuing* contributions, ideas, difference.

Table 4.2 provides a structure within which team members can review their individual understanding of others' knowledge, skills and job roles. It also provides a format for pooling and comparing understanding in order to identify areas in which there is a need for more clarity.

When to use it

Teams can use this at any stage in their development. It is our experience that teams are often working with assumptions around roles that can mean duplication of effort, things getting missed or rising frustration in individuals who are not using their skills and knowledge. Or efforts are not being appreciated, which in turn has a negative impact on team dynamics and motivation.

Suggestions for use in practice

- Create a list of team members or, if there are more than 10, the names of different professional groups within your team.
- Write the names of the team members or professional groups in the first column of the grid.
- Ask all team members to complete the grid.
- When all team members have completed the grid, use the information provided to identify areas in which greater clarity is required, and to design ways in which this can be achieved.

Table 4.2: Role clarity review grid

Names of individuals or professional groups (or other teams)	How much do you know about this individual or group's job content?				How much do you know about this individual or group's knowledge, skills and ways of working?				How well does this individual or group use your knowledge and skills?			
	Nothing	Very little	A fair amount	A great deal	Nothing	Very little	A fair amount	A great deal	Very poorly	To a limited extent	Well	Very well

Source: Aston OD (2007)

Creative thinking: De Bono's 'Thinking hats'

Much is written in the literature about the ability of effective teams to be creative. Creativity is not necessarily about completely new ideas, but it is 'connecting and rearranging of knowledge – in the minds of people who will allow them to think flexibly – to generate new, often surprising ideas that others judge to be useful' (Plsek, 1997, p 27). If *creativity* is the new idea, then *innovation* is the implementation of this or the way of working in order to *improve* service delivery.

Creativity remains an idealised concept unless organisations and managers create conditions where it can truly flourish. People need time and space in order to be able to think differently, which usually has resource implications (either in terms of time or money). One tool that can be used to aid practical, creative thinking is de Bono's (1985) 'Thinking hats' technique (see Figure 4.2).

What does it seek to explore?

The 'Thinking hats' tool is made up of six different hats that represent six different ways of thinking about an issue, which de Bono called 'lateral thinking'. We do not often recognise that we are thinking about a problem in a particular way. If we do not like something or are negative about an issue, we may not recognise that we are conceptualising this in a pessimistic manner. By hearing different viewpoints, or thinking about an issue from a different perspective, this should become apparent. When discussing issues, one viewpoint will often have a tendency to dominate, but using this technique means that emotions, hard facts and the positives and negatives associated with an issue are all given a hearing.

When to use it

The possibilities are numerous, but include when a team needs to consider a new approach to service delivery, or a new approach to any of its systems, tasks or processes. It could also be helpful if the team is stuck on an issue, where taking time to explore it in a structured and non-emotive way (albeit acknowledging emotion) could be helpful. We have also used it with teams who have undergone significant learning events and post-serious untoward incidents.

Suggestions for use in practice

Teams use this tool to consider 'one hat' at a time and to think through the implications of this factor. Issues need different approaches, and for some it is useful to start with (and clarify) the facts before working systematically through the hats presented in Figure 4.2. It can often be a useful exercise to try and think about such an issue with a 'yellow hat', and ponder all the potential positives that are associated with it. Similarly, when we have a good idea it is easy to get carried away. It may be useful in these situations to put on the 'black hat', and seriously think through any potential negatives that might be associated with this idea.

Figure 4.2: De Bono's 'Thinking hats'

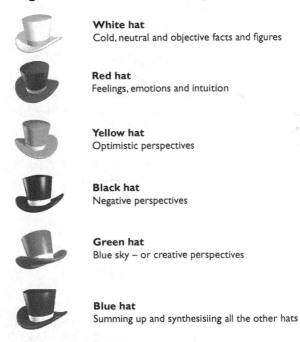

White hat
Cold, neutral and objective facts and figures

Red hat
Feelings, emotions and intuition

Yellow hat
Optimistic perspectives

Black hat
Negative perspectives

Green hat
Blue sky – or creative perspectives

Blue hat
Summing up and synthesiiing all the other hats

Source: de Bono (1985)

Using the de Bono tool is one way of hearing a range of voices and issues that may otherwise be subsumed in discussions around complex issues. However, simply deciding on the course of action for the future is not quite the end of the process. Without organisations and line managers giving sufficient freedom to individuals and teams to make decisions over an issue, they can do all the creative thinking they want but will not be able to act on it. This is illustrative of the way in which many of the factors that make up real teams are interlinked.

Communication and cooperation: The SBAR approach

Communication has been mentioned frequently throughout this book, and it is a very real obstacle that many teams encounter problems with. One model increasingly used by teams in a variety of care environments to better communicate is the SBAR model.

What does it seek to explore?

The SBAR model seeks to give a predictable structure to communication. This has been standard procedure within the aviation and nuclear industries, and is increasingly used in some healthcare settings. The letters in acronym are described as follows:

- *Situation:* a concise statement of the problem
- *Background:* pertinent and brief information related to the situation
- *Assessment:* analysis and consideration of options
- *Recommendation:* action/recommendations.

The model is based on the principles of the assertion cycle (see Figure 4.3). One of the difficulties of communication is its influence by social processes. Individuals may feel constrained by issues of hierarchy or power and unable to state a problem and secure an answer. Often people speak indirectly and hint at the existence of a problem, hoping that colleagues pick up on this. But there are clearly quite large risk implications here. The assertion cycle states a problem politely and persistently until an answer is received. If all members of a team are used to using this approach, then if an individual states 'I need to see you now', their colleague knows that this cannot wait. Although this clearly has applications within critical care contexts, it is equally applicable to all care settings.

When to use it

We know from the literature that things often go wrong at the boundaries of care, so this model can be used (and is being used) to structure the handover of information across departments, agencies, teams, or from one shift to another. Additionally, as in the example below (see Box 4.2), it can be used when asking for help or advice about a changing situation. We talked in Chapter 3 about the impact of agency staff and changing medical working hours, meaning that people do not often have the relationships with each other they might have had historically. A model such as SBAR, which is used by everyone in a given area, can help overcome the barriers of not knowing each other, and helps people to think through how to structure their communication to get their message across and to be clear about actions, in a clear and succinct way.

Suggestions for use in practice

Haig et al (2006) demonstrate how this model has been successfully used in teams in North America and Australia to improve communication by structuring conversations within and across teams, and Box 4.2 illustrates how the tool could be used in practice.

Box 4.2: Using the SBAR approach

The outlining *situation* should pick up any potential difficulties with different professional approaches to language and narrative. Individuals should clearly and briefly state the problem in a way that others understand. The information shared at this stage should cover exactly what the problem is: "Dr Khan, I'm calling about Mrs Weston, who is experiencing increased anxiety."

The *background* provides information that is succinct, pertinent and factual. What were the circumstances leading up to this problem? "She is a 74-year-old woman who is receiving medication for anxiety, but is getting much worse."

With *assessment* the conversation moves on to an analysis of the current situation and leads to what you think the problem is: "She is constantly 'phoning about problems and has not left the house for two weeks."

The conversation ends on *recommendation*, where specific actions are outlined and agreed on clearly. This is the area that often fails in communication processes, as different parties are not clear about the action and priority of the next steps: "I need you to see her today at your outpatient clinic. She needs her medication reviewing and referral to a psychologist."
Source: Based on Leonard et al (2004)

Figure 4.3: The assertion cycle

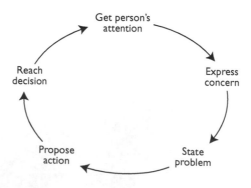

Team meetings: Thinking Environment® meeting

While meetings are a constant feature of organisational life, many people struggle to handle the dynamics and emotions that can be displayed when groups come together. But meetings can tap into a rich source of knowledge and expertise, and it is important to remember that individuals struggle to engage with things they have not been part of exploring.

The Thinking Environment meeting, developed from Nancy Kline's research (2009), is a structured and effective way of tapping into the resourcefulness of team members, and having effective, valuable meetings where issues are explored and ways forward are clear. Her research has identified tangible benefits from using Thinking Environment tools, including the following:

- A company rescued a £200 million product in 45 minutes.
- A government agency saved 62% of senior management time over six to twelve months.
- A medical team saved 44% of the cost of each decision.
- A hospital moved in nine months from 1 to 4 stars.
- A telecommunications company saved 30 days of work in 40 minutes.

The Thinking Environment meeting structure also contains these important features:

- It is effective for any kind of meeting (business, planning, strategy, creative thinking etc).
- It allows for a meeting of many agenda items of many kinds.
- Each agenda item is in the form of a question.
- It can take place around a table, as usual.
- It allows for decision-making and action agreements.
- It can replace completely the usual, less productive and less participative meeting framework most teams use.

What does it seek to explore?

The way people *behave* with each other actually determines the quality of their *thinking*. The tool is based on the 10 components of the Thinking Environment that create conditions where people can think clearly:

- *Attention:* listening with palpable respect, with interest in where the thinker will go next, and without interruption.
- *Equality:* treating each other as thinking peers giving equal turns and attention, keeping agreements and boundaries.
- *Ease:* offering freedom from internal rush or urgency.
- *Appreciation:* offering genuine acknowledgement of a person's qualities; practising a 5:1 ratio of appreciation to criticism.
- *Encouragement:* giving courage to go to the unpopular or cutting edge of ideas by moving beyond internal competition.
- *Feelings:* allowing sufficient emotional release to restore thinking.
- *Information:* supplying the facts; dismantling denial.
- *Diversity:* welcoming divergent thinking and diverse group identities.
- *Incisive questions:* removing assumptions that limit our ability to think for ourselves clearly and creatively.
- *Place:* creating a physical environment that says to people, 'You matter'.

Source: © Nancy Kline (2010)

When to use it

When individuals or the team have problems and puzzles and dilemmas they need to understand and explore further.

Suggestions for use in practice

This offers a very structured way of meeting. It is important that the process is adhered to, which demands discipline from everyone. Working in a clockwise direction, people are invited to contribute in turn, as set out below (see Box 4.3). This stops people talking over each other, contributing randomly, and starting other conversations. The underlying premise is that the structure and discipline of listening and contributing help the person who has introduced the issue to think clearly and to be able to access everyone else's best thinking.

Box 4.3: The Thinking Environment® meeting

- *The opening round:* Going around the group, the chair of the meeting gives everyone a turn to answer positively-focused questions, such as: 'What is going well in your work at the moment?' 'What do you think we as a team (board, organisation, etc) are currently doing well?'
- *The agenda:* The chair confirms the agenda and identifies the first item for discussion. The agenda may include a presentation, clarification round, agenda item question, open discussion round etc.
- *Additional processes:* Thinking pairs (the team break into pairs to think about a point under discussion); dialogue; removing assumptions; decision and action.
- *Burning issues:* When the meeting is almost at an end, the chair asks each person, 'Is there a burning issue that you think we should address at another time?'
- *The closing round:* Any concerns should have been handled or mentioned by this point, so the closing can be wholly positive. The chair asks everyone to answer positively-reflective questions, such as 'What do you think went well in the meeting?', and ideally, 'What one quality do you respect in the colleague sitting to your right?'

Source: © Nancy Kline (2010)

Team effectiveness: The five dysfunctions

We have seen throughout this book that there is a real cost to the quality and safety of services where teams are ineffective. We have chosen to bring to life the concept of a dysfunctional team with a model that makes intuitive sense and integrates themes introduced throughout this book.

What does it seek to explore?

The five dysfunctions of a team model described by Lencioni (2002) (see Figure 4.4) tries to get to grips with the issue of why so many teams struggle. It is presented as a hierarchy, with interdependencies between each level. Absence of trust is the foundation that leads to the potential for more dysfunction to develop if it is not present, respected and nurtured.

The five dysfunctions are as follows:

- *Absence of trust:* this relates not just to individuals trusting each other, but also reluctance to be seen as vulnerable. If individuals are unable (or feel unable) to be open with one another about their weaknesses and mistakes, then it is impossible to build a foundation for trust to develop. This also returns to an earlier message in the book, that people need to trust each other in order to take risks and to improve services through innovation. Lack of stability is often the reason that people struggle to develop trusting relationships with each other as they do not know each other and so cannot sufficiently predict what the future actions of their partners will be.
- *Fear of conflict:* this is at the heart of many of the problems in dysfunctional teams. People are afraid to, or do not know how to, manage conflict, and it is therefore often left to fester and grow into something destructive that has a major impact on a range of people. Conflict is often seen negatively rather than as a difference of opinion between two parties that needs working through. Avoiding conflict may mean that there is not a culture of challenge and passionate debate in teams (elements that are positively associated with safety). Investment in conflict resolution skills for staff working at all levels of systems should be a major priority for all organisations in health and social care.

- *Lack of commitment:* individuals not committing to decisions subsequently undermine decisions the team has made.
- *Avoidance of accountability:* this is the reluctance to hold people to account for their practice, behaviours and actions that might be counterproductive to the effectiveness of the team.
- *Inattention to results:* this occurs when people put their individual needs, wishes and interests above the collective goals of the team.

When to use it

Teams can use this as a framework at any stage in their development to consider how they are functioning. It can be particularly helpful if something has gone wrong in the team, or if the team has had feedback that it is not performing as expected. Or it can be used as part of a development plan that looks at team strengths – and the team needs to decide how it will sustain and further develop its effectiveness.

Suggestions for use in practice

If people are largely familiar with the five stages of the model and the meaning and interpretation of each dysfunction, these can be used to analyse the team (either alone, or with others) to explore perceptions, reality and feelings about each dimension, and then to decide on any action that needs to be taken. We have, on occasion, suggested that team members read Lencioni (2002) (it will take about two hours) in advance of a team session. Reframing issues through considering the experiences of another team (in this case that of the team in Lencioni, 2002) can provide a creative technique to open dialogues within teams of their own practice.

Figure 4.4: The five dysfunctions of a team

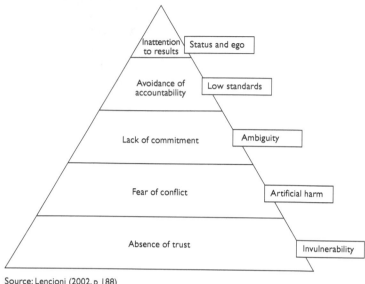

Source: Lencioni (2002, p 188)

Tools and frameworks for organisations

Organisations have a critical role in creating conditions where teams can flourish, and it is essential to create conditions whereby teamworking and interprofessional working can happen in a meaningful way. There is a much greater emphasis on culture in this second edition of the book, which is reflective of learning and incidents that have happened globally over the last few years. Here we introduce a tool that offers ways of considering culture for organisations (and teams).

Mapping organisation culture: The cultural web

The cultural web is a much-used idea from Johnson et al (2008) that focuses on a series of elements that it is argued make up the feel of the work environment. By analysing these different behavioural, physical and symbolic manifestations of culture, it is suggested that you can gain a perspective on your organisation's culture and have an insight into what is and is not working

What does it seek to explore?

Johnson et al (2008) introduce seven areas that link together to form a web (see Figure 4.5).

They argue that physically mapping organisation culture can:

- help to question things that are usually taken for granted;
- identify barriers to progression and change;
- facilitate consideration of the alignment of culture with existing strategy;
- provide a basis for examining what changes need to occur to deliver a new strategy.

The elements are:

- *The paradigm*: taken-for-granted assumptions form the core of an organisation's culture.
- *Stories:* the past events and people talked about inside and outside the organisation. These stories are typically about successes, things that went wrong, heroes, villains and mavericks (who deviate from the norm). They can be a way of letting people know what is important in a given organisation.
- *Symbols:* these are the visual representation of an organisation which can include objects, events, acts and people that create, convey or maintain meaning over their functional purpose.
- *Power structures:* the pockets of real power in the organisation. The key is that these people have the greatest amount of influence on decisions, operations and strategic direction.
- *Organisational structures:* this is likely to reflect power and show important roles and relationships.
- *Control systems:* measurements and reward systems that emphasise what is important in an organisation.

- *Rituals and routines:* routines are 'the way we do things around here', on a day-to-day basis. They may have a long history, and at their best they can help the organisation to function, but they can represent a taken-for-grantedness (see Chapter 3) about how things should happen, which can be hard to change. Rituals are about activities or events that emphasise, and at times reinforce, what is especially important in the culture.

Figure 4.5: The cultural web of an organisation

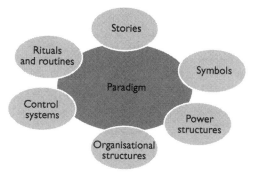

Source: Johnson et al (2008)

When to use it

When a group wants to understand culture. This may be in response to feedback, an incident or perhaps just taking stock of how things are.

Suggestions for use in practice

Take time to consider these areas. How would you (or your team) complete the circles? Use the definitions of each area in the section above, 'What does it seek to explore?', to help guide thinking and exploration. We have worked with board members to undertake this exercise, and then introduced the board to people working at other levels of the organisation who have also completed the tool. The ensuing discussion around why people see and experience things differently was illuminating for all.

Assessing the effectiveness of teamworking: Aston Team Performance Inventory

Organisations need to invest in tools, processes and systems that give teams the information they need to understand their effectiveness. Frameworks that help teams to understand their effectiveness are essential if they are to objectively understand their performance and to take responsibility for it. There are many tools that claim to measure effectiveness, but we have chosen to introduce the Aston Team Performance Inventory (ATPI) because it offers an evidence-based and comprehensive assessment of the team's potential to be effective (see Figure 4.6).

Figure 4.6: Aston Team Performance Inventory

Inputs	Processes	Outputs
Team task design Effort and skills Organisational support	**Team processes** Objectives Reflexivity Participation Task focus Team conflict Creativity and innovation	Individual satisfaction Attachment Team effectiveness Long-term relationships
	Leadership Leading Managing Coaching	

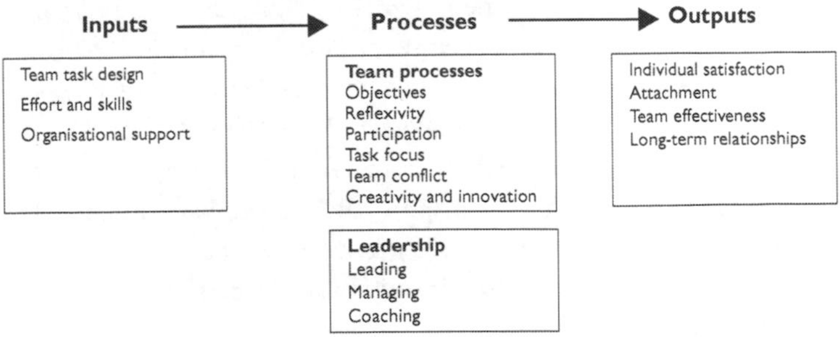

Source: Aston OD (2008)

What does it seek to explore?

Based on years of research and learning (much of it in health and social care), the ATPI is an input-process-output (IPO) model (see Chapter 2), which also has the added dimension of leadership. Eighteen sub-areas bring these four dimensions to life, and team members are asked to rate the effectiveness and functioning of their team on a scale of 1-5. The comprehensive report shows mean responses, as well as the range of responses, so people can see where views and perceptions differ. A shortened version of this tool has also been developed (the Aston Real Team Profile), and a suite of development tools based on the diagnostic frameworks is successfully used in many organisations across the UK and Europe.

When to use it

Teams could use this tool as part of a tailored development programme or in preparation for an away day in order to 'take the temperature of the team'. It could be useful when something has gone wrong, or perhaps when organisation metrics are indicating that there may be a problem in a team (for example, rising number of incidents, complaints, sickness, absence, problems recruiting, high turnover). It may be useful when a new leader is in post to understand the current effectiveness of teamworking or alternatively, perhaps, six months after the team leader has been in post. It can also be helpful where teams have integrated to understand how team members see the working of the team. It is also used as part of tailored team-based working and leadership programmes, commissioned by organisations.

Suggestions for use in practice

Once the tool has been completed it is important that the team come together to review the results. Data isn't attributable to individuals, so people should feel safe to complete it. It does show the range of responses and it can be helpful for teams to explore why individuals may see things so differently. It can be set up so that in addition to the one overall team report, there are subgroup reports. This can be especially helpful if teams are keen to explore the experiences of different groups, for example, different professions, full or part-time staff, or qualified or unqualified staff. Organisations can commission composite reports, so they can see and learn from the themes across teams, which could contribute to their organisational development or service improvement strategy.

Tools and frameworks for partnerships

We now turn our attention to partnership working across agencies and teams, as this is another key contextual factor, particularly for inter-agency teams.

Partnerships: The working inventory

What does it seek to explore?

The effective partnership working inventory (West and Markiewicz, 2006) aims to measure seven dimensions that are known from research to be critical to the development of effective partnership working – both in multidisciplinary and multiagency teams (illustrated in Figure 4.7). These seven dimensions are further developed in Box 4.4, which gives a list illustrating how a partnership might check their degree of effectiveness against each of these different competencies.

When to use it

It could be useful to use this at the beginning of a new partnership as a framework to guide elements and processes that need to be in place. Timing is always key, and the partnership itself could best decide when would be good time to use it as an evaluation of current perceptions of working.

Suggestions for use in practice

Partnerships can use this to assess which domains they are operating effectively within and which need further development. As this expanded list suggests, teams may need to complete multiple versions of this in respect of the different links they have in terms of the team itself, its own organisation(s) and wider partners. Readers of this book might wish to use this to highlight any areas in which their team needs to develop, and then use the tools offered in this chapter to aid this process.

Figure 4.7: Seven dimensions of effective partnership working

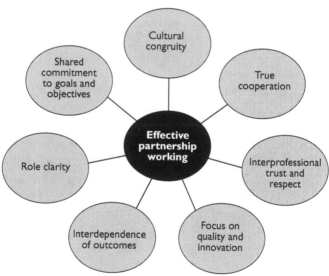

Source: West and Markiewicz (2006)

Box 4.4: Dimensions of effective partnership working

Shared commitment to goals and objectives

All partnership members:

- are clear about their own home team and organisation's goals
- are clear about the partnership's goals
- believe that the goals of the partnership are valuable
- enter into the partnership willingly.

Interdependence of outcomes

All partnership members believe:

- their home team, organisation and partnership's goals are interdependent
- innovation is required to achieve these goals
- the skills and experience brought to the partnership by all the different partners are essential to success.

Role clarity

All partnership members:

- understand their own and each other's role within the partnership
- ensure that power and status relationships are agreed and described
- work constructively to resolve conflicts that may arise about status or role.

Cultural congruity

All partnership members:

- understand differences between cultures across home teams or across organisational cultures
- spend time to develop effective processes for working together
- regularly review working and interpersonal relationships.

Focus on quality and innovation

All partnership members:

- demonstrate a concern for quality that is focused on the aims of the partnership

- encourage positive challenging and regular constructive debate about working practices
- share learning from errors or mistakes
- provide practical support for innovation in working practices.

True cooperation

All partnership members:
- define the requirements for effective partnership working
- design integrated policies and working practices
- provide training for partnership working at all levels of the partnership
- ensure effective communication processes exist and are managed effectively.

Interprofessional trust and respect

In relation to other professional groups within the partnership, all individuals:
- understand the professional roles of each group
- understand the different ways of working traditionally adopted by each group
- use positive language to describe the role and contribution of others
- provide constructive feedback to colleagues from all professional groups.

Source: Adapted from West and Markiewicz (2006)

Integrated care arrangements: Development Model for Integrated Care

Understanding context can help to identify factors that will support or prevent interprofessional teamworking and the potential contribution that teams can make to broader aspirations for greater collaboration. Many of the tools that are available look at particular elements of collaboration and/or are focused on the more strategic level. The Development Model for Integrated Care (DMIC) provides a holistic perspective and is targeted at service delivery. It was originally developed in the Netherlands but is now being used in North America and elsewhere in Europe, and has been deployed within a range of integrated care services including community mental health and older people's services, cardiology and neurology (Minkman et al, 2009).

What does it seek to explore?

The DMIC identifies nine dimensions that are key to integrated care. These dimensions (or clusters) are further broken down into activities (or elements) that can help realise these in practice (see Table 4.3). The model also recognises that there are stages in development of an integrated care services and that the dimensions will be gradually introduced during implementation. The stages are: (1) initiative and design; (2) experiment and execution; (3) expansion and monitoring; and (4) consolidation and transformation.

When to use it

The DMIC can be administered through surveys and as the basis for interviews and focus groups discussions. It can be helpful at all stages of the development and implementation of an interprofessional team, from initially deciding if the context will be supportive of such a team being introduced to reviewing progress in achieving the expected impacts and supporting team processes.

Suggestions for use in practice

Along with other such audit-based tools, DMIC is best used as part of an ongoing service improvement process. Gathering the data will by itself encourage team members and stakeholders in reflecting on the purpose, functioning and impact of the team and the service that it sits within, and the analysis of findings can then help to identify what is working well and what needs to be addressed. Repeating the data gathering on a periodic basis helps to review what has been achieved and the next priorities for action.

Table 4.3: Development Model for Integrated Care elements of integration

Patient-family-centred care	Care is focused on the needs of service users, patients and families, and there is good communication between them and care providers
Delivery system	Agreements are in place between partners on care pathways and coordinating mechanisms are available for patients and service users with complex needs
Performance management	A holistic framework is in place that gathers data on outcomes for patients and service users, experience of accessing the service, organisational outcomes and financial performance
Quality of care	Evidence-based interprofessional care is provided in response to patient-family needs and preferences
Result-focused learning	A supportive culture that promotes interprofessional working through defining clear goals, identifying bottlenecks and gaps in care, and exchanging knowledge and performance in an open atmosphere. Incentives are used to reward improved results
Interprofessional teamwork	There are 'real' interprofessional teams whose work fits into overall care pathways
Roles and tasks	There is clarity about the expertise, roles and tasks of the professionals and agencies involved
Commitment	There is commitment from the individual professionals to the defined objectives they intend to contribute, and they have skills and knowledge in interprofessional working
Transparent entrepreneurship	There is the opportunity for leaders within the service to respond innovatively to opportunities and challenges, and there are financial arrangements that encourage organisations to take and share risks

Source: Minkman et al (2009)

This chapter has sought to provide an overview of some key frameworks, models and tools that may help to develop and enhance understanding of effective teamworking. Central to this process is the need to take time to reflect on what the issues really are (the what) and then to further reflect on the best way forward (the how and the who). Indeed, this is a key message of this entire book, that partnerships need to be clear about what they are trying to achieve, and use these aims to inform the structure and processes of subsequent relationships. All too often teams (understandably) get wrapped up with the way in which things currently do or do not work, without looking above the immediate context and seeing what could be. As suggested in Chapter 1, real teams have a clear focus on what it is they are trying to achieve by working together. By bearing these aims in mind and employing some of the frameworks and models outlined in this chapter, teams should be able to work together more effectively.

Reflective exercises

1. Take time to reflect on your personal team contribution – use the questions in Box 4.1 to guide your thinking.
2. Think about a decision you have to take, or an issue that you are working on and apply de Bono's 'Thinking hats' (Figure 4.2). Start with the facts ('white hat') and work through the remaining colours.
3. Use the SBAR model (Box 4.2) to think about a recent handover. How clearly was information communicated, and were the final actions understood by all parties?
4. We have argued throughout the book that real teams need to meet, and those meetings need to work well to include the thoughts and ideas of the diverse members. How could you use the structure and processes in the Thinking Environment meeting (see Box 4.3) to further improve the quality and participation of your team meetings?
5. Think about Lencioni's model of a dysfunctional team (see Figure 4.4). What does your team do well and not so well?
6. Reflect on the elements of the cultural web (Figure 4.5) – how would you and your team complete the circles?
7. Consider another team or organisation that you are working collaboratively with, and reflect on the dimensions of the effective partnership working inventory (Figure 4.7 and Box 4.4).
8. If your team works within an integrated care initiative, what stage of development would you consider that you have reached? How would you assess your strengths against the nine dimensions of the DMIC (Table 4.3)?

Further reading and resources

References relating to key texts underpinning the chapter can be found in the final References section at the end of the book. In addition:

- The work of Aston Organisation Development (Aston OD) is built around a strong belief that effective teamworking is key to the delivery of high quality and compassionate health and social care. The team works across the NHS and with others who recognise the positive impact of high performing teams on patient and organisational outcomes. They aim to help organisations build good team and interteam working. Their suite of research-based tools are widely used by service improvement, OD and learning development practitioners who want to assess, develop and monitor the performance of teams but struggle with limited resources and constant change: www.astonod.com

- The Belbin team roles website has a wealth of tools, information and resources (many of them free) about how to work with Belbin team roles in practice: www.belbin.com. Explanation of the team roles can be found at: www.youtube.com/watch?v=9M0AI3Oi0-8&feature=youtu.be

- Accessible information about coaching and mentoring may be found at the Coaching & Mentoring Network. This site is primarily aimed at coaches and people looking for coaches, but has a good resource centre that is freely available and contains full text articles, case studies and up-to-date news: www.coachingnetwork.org.uk

- The European Mentoring & Coaching Council (EMCC) UK is part of the Europe-wide EMCC, which exists to promote good practice and the expectation of good practice in mentoring and coaching across Europe. EMCC UK is an independent, impartial and non-profit-making organisation. The website contains a wealth of information and signposts resources: www.emccouncil.org/

- The Canadian Patient Safety Institute (CPSI) has over 15 years of experience in safety leadership and implementing programmes to enhance safety in every part of the healthcare continuum. A federally funded not-for-profit organisation, CPSI offers products and programmes focused on four priority areas: medication safety, surgical care safety, infection prevention and control, and home care safety. CPSI is developing a Canadian Framework for Teamwork and Communication to help healthcare providers and organisations integrate tools and resources into practice: www.patientsafetyinstitute.ca/en/toolsResources/teamworkCommunication/Pages/default.aspx

- The Chartered Institute of Personnel and Development (CIPD) is the UK's leading professional body for those involved in the management and development of people. Many selected resources, papers and tools are free: www.cipd.co.uk

- The Human Resources for Health (HRC) Global Resource Center is a digital global library focused on developing countries: www.hrhresourcecenter.org/

- The Institute for Healthcare Improvement (IHI) aims to improve health and healthcare worldwide. Its comprehensive website has a wealth of resources and tools (including audio and video programmes) to help it achieve its aim. We have signposted links to tools about structured communication and safety that have been a focus of the last two chapters:

  - SBAR toolkit: www.ihi.org/resources/pages/tools/sbartoolkit.aspx

  - Structured communication and psychological safety in healthcare: www.ihi.org/resources/Pages/AudioandVideo/WIHISBARStructuredCommunicationandPsychological SafetyinHealthCare.aspx

- The Integrated Team Monitoring and Assessment (ITMA) tool is freely available for integrated teams in order to provide a relatively simple and cost-effective way of assessing the effectiveness of teamworking. It enables a rapid appraisal of the 'health' of a team, and identifies areas of difficulty covering both internal functioning and external factors, thereby enabling a focus on remedial action commensurate with the significance of the problems: www.wales.nhs.uk/sitesplus/documents/829/ICN%20Integrated%20Team%20Monitoring%20and%20Assessment.doc

- The Mind Tools website has a range of resources and materials to increase productivity, improve management and leadership skills, and support organisational development initiatives. People can access and learn useful career skills for free, and can also learn new skills through their Facebook, Twitter and LinkedIn pages, and with their YouTube channel: www.mindtools.com/pages/article/newTMM_84.htm
- Nancy Kline's Time to Think website has a range of case studies, research, references and assessment tools all created to help people to consider and improve the quality of thinking and listening: www.timetothink.com/
- Paul Plesk's site, DirectedCreativity.com™, has a wealth of tools and information around the issue of creativity: www.directedcreativity.com
- Professional organisations have websites with a wealth of tools, links and signposts to other resources research and support. For example, the Royal College of Nursing in the UK produced Developing and sustaining effective teams with the former NHS Institute for Innovation and Improvement: www2.rcn.org.uk/__data/assets/pdf_file/0003/78735/003115.pdf
- The World Health Organization (WHO) has developed a safety curriculum with a range of topics that contribute to patient safety. Being an effective team player is an essential part of the curriculum: www.who.int/patientsafety/education/curriculum/who_mc_topic-4.pdf

5

Recommendations for policy and practice

Ultimately, the evidence, questions, summaries, learning and frameworks set out in this book lead us to make a series of practical recommendations and potential warnings, both for policy and for practice.

For policy-makers

- There is a need to consider the implications for existing teams and services when they exhort new teams or style of working. Creating new teams in any area will affect existing teams, their working practices and relationships, and may hinder the development of practice as people struggle to differentiate roles and boundaries.
- Measures of teams in organisations are sometimes only built around their existence, not around their effectiveness; this perhaps adds to cynicism around rhetoric, as opposed to commitment, to teamworking.
- Although teamworking may be helpful in a number of ways, it is not a default position that will solve all difficulties. Teams need real tasks and a real need to work together in order to be effective. Simply ordering more of certain types of teams will not overcome the difficulties that health and social care communities face.
- National policy needs to send out stronger messages about how organisations need to make investments in enhancing and sustaining teamworking, rather than just one-off training.

- There is a real need to have some stability in the system. Improvement in services is about doing something differently. To do this, people need to take risks and they will not feel safe to do so until there is a climate of mutual trust and respect, which takes time to develop.
- There is an increasing tendency within commissioning to design specific care pathways (that is, for certain conditions or client groups), rather than commissioning particular professional services (for example, district nursing services). The implication of this is that there will be a greater demand to work across boundaries and for individual professionals to work as teams. World class commissioning should demand that appropriate support and development needs to be made available to support professionals and teamworking in these roles.

For local organisations and front-line services

- Do not underestimate the power and importance of teamworking. There is a tendency in health and social care settings not to prioritise team development, as care inputs are seen as more immediately important. However, team development and teamworking do have real implications for the quality of services delivered, particularly within inter-agency settings. At the same time people need to be encouraged to think about whether the task at hand really needs a team – there is a need for teams to tackle real issues as conflict is draining and has an impact on everyone.
- Teams really do need time to be teams. Just putting everyone together and expecting them to work effectively without ever being able to meet, debate and explore will not work. Evidence is very clear about the importance of creating conditions to develop reflexivity and the subsequent relationship to improved innovation and quality of services. Overt organisational commitment to this is crucial. We need clear messages from leaders in organisations that time for teams is valuable and supported.
- New ways of working and the associated new design of facilities can mean that traditional ways of meeting are getting harder. If teams

are to be effective, they need to be able to meet, and they need somewhere to do so!

- If there are to be changes around teamworking or integration, leaders must take time to find out about how people are currently working. Much more partnership and teamworking is taking place than is recognised. The work of practitioners and existing teams needs to be valued.

- The increasing development towards the commissioning of care pathways as opposed to the commissioning of professional services will see the need to work across boundaries and teamworking increase. As a result, the key issues and frameworks in this book will become even more important over time.

- Research tells us that middle managers are under the most stress, and there are often no easy answers to many of the complex problems and issues that they are facing. However, investment in development in the form of mentoring, coaching and learning sets may provide valuable returns.

- If organisations are to hold teams accountable and responsible, they need to have autonomy and authority. If teams are to be held to account for their actions, they also need some freedom over how they operate.

So, finally, there really are no great secrets about teamworking, but different knowledge levels, skills, intuition and experiences make it a contested arena. It is not a panacea for all situations, but an area that needs real commitment, investment and curiosity. The conditions for the nurturing of teams are crucial. Inhospitable conditions will mean that they wither and fail to grow. Some commitment to create the right conditions will see some growth, but real commitment to creating the right environment will likely see teams flourish, unleashing potential and energy that will take them in often surprising directions in their quest to develop innovative services and care (see Figure 5.1).

Figure 5.1: Nurturing the effectiveness of teams

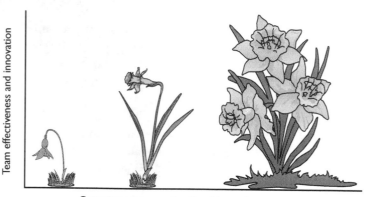

Team effectiveness and innovation

Commitment to creating the right environment

References

6, P., Glasby, J. and Lester, H. (2007) 'Incremental change without policy learning: explaining information rejection in English mental health services', *Journal of Comparative Policy Analysis*, vol 9, pp 21-46.

6, P., Leat, D., Seltzer, K. and Stoker, G. (2002) *Towards holistic governance: The new reform agenda*, New York: Palgrave.

Allen, N. and Hecht, T. (2004) 'The "romance" of teams: toward an understanding of its psychological underpinnings and implications', *Journal of Occupational and Organizational Psychology*, vol 77, pp 439-61.

Appelbaum, E. and Batt, R. (1994) *The new American workplace*, Ithaca, NY: ILR Press.

Aston OD (Organisation Development) (nd) 'Aston Team Performance Toolkit' (www.astonod.com/team-tools/aston-team-performance-toolkit/).

Audit Commission (1992) *Homeward bound: A new course for community health*, London: HMSO.

Baggott, R. (2010) *Public health: Policy and politics* (2nd edn), Basingstoke: Palgrave Macmillan.

Ballatt, J. and Campling, P. (2011) *Intelligent kindness: Reforming the culture of healthcare*, London: RCPsych Publications.

Balloch, S. and Taylor, M. (2001) *Partnership working: Policy and practice*, Bristol: Policy Press.

Barrett, G., Sellman, D. and Thomas, J. (eds) (2005) *Interprofessional working in health and social care: Professional perspectives*, Basingstoke: Palgrave.

Belbin, M. (2000) *Beyond the team*, Oxford: Butterworth-Heinemann.

Bilodeau, K., Dubois, S. and Pepin, J. (2014) 'Interprofessional patient-centred practice in oncology teams: utopia or reality?', *Journal of Interprofessional Care*, vol 29, no 2, pp 106-12.

BMA (British Medical Association) (1974) *Primary health care teams*, London: BMA.

Borrill, C., Carletta, J., Carter, A., Dawson, J., Garrod, S., Rees, A. et al (2001) *The effectiveness of health care teams in the National Health Service*, Aston: Aston Centre for Health Service Organization Research.

Bostock, L., Bairstow, S., Fish, S. and Macleod, F. (2005) *Managing risk and minimising mistakes to services for children and families*, London: Social Care Institute for Excellence.

Boston, R. (2014) *ARC leadership: From surviving to thriving in a complex world*, London: LeaderSpace.

Bridges, J. and Fuller, A. (2014) 'Creating learning environments for compassionate care: a programme to promote compassionate care by health and social care teams', *International journal of Older people Nursing*, vol 10, pp 48-58.

Briggs Myers, I. (revised by K. Kirby and K.D. Myers) (2000) *An introduction to Type®: A guide to understanding your results on the Myers-Briggs Type indicator* (6th edn), London: Oxford Psychologists Press.

Briggs Myers, I. and Myers, P.B. (1995) *Gifts differing: Understanding personality type*, Mountain View, CA: Davies-Black Publishing (CPP, Inc).

British Medical Journal (2004) 'Ombudsman', vol 328, p 10.

Buchanan, D. (2011) 'Reflections: good practice, not rocket science – understanding failures to change after extreme events', *Journal of Change Management*, vol 11, no 3, pp 273-88.

Burgess, N. and Radnor, Z. (2013) 'Evaluating Lean in healthcare', *International Journal of Health Care Quality Assurance*, vol 26, issue 3, pp 220-35.

Buttigieg, S.C., Cassar, V. and Scully, J. (2013) 'From words to action: Visibility of management in supporting interdisciplinary team working in an acute rehabilitative geriatric hospital', *Journal of Health Organization and Management*, vol 27, issue 5, pp 618-45.

Butow, P., Mikhail, M., Jefford, M. and King, M. on behalf of the Psycho-Oncology Co-operative Research Group (2011) 'From inside the bubble: migrants' perceptions of communication with the cancer team', *Support Care Cancer*, vol 19, pp 281-90.

Cass, A., Lowell, A., Christie, M., Snelling, P., Flack, M., Marrnganyin, B. and Brown, I. (2002) 'Sharing the true stories: improving communication between Aboriginal patients and healthcare workers', *The Medical Journal of Australia*, vol 176, no 10, pp 466-70.

Cameron, A. and Lart, R. (2003) 'Factors promoting and obstacles hindering joint working: a systematic review of the research evidence', *Journal of Integrated Care*, vol 11, issue 2, pp 9-17.

Carpenter, J. and Dickinson, H. (2016) *Interprofessional education and training* (2nd edn), Better Partnership Working series, Bristol: Policy Press.

Cheng, C., Bartram, T., Karimi, L. and Leggatt, S. (2013) 'The role of team climate in the management of emotional labour: implications for nurse retention', *Journal of Advanced Nursing*, vol 69, no 12, pp 2812-25.

CIPD (Chartered Institute of Personnel and Development) (2013a) *Real-life leaders: Closing the knowing-doing gap*, Research report, September, London: CIPD.

CIPD (2013b) *Employee outlook: Focus on trust in leaders*, Research report, Autumn, London: CIPD.

Cohen, S. and Bailey, D. (1997) 'What makes teams work: group effectiveness research from the shop floor to the executive suite', *Journal of Management*, vol 23, pp 239-90.

Cook, D.A., Hatala, R., Brydges, R., Zendejas, B., Szostek, J.H., Wang, A.T. et al (2011) 'Technology-enhanced simulation for health professions education: a systematic review and meta-analysis', *JAMA*, vol 306, no 9, pp 978-88.

Cornwall, J. (2011) 'Care and compassion in the NHS', Blog on The King's Fund website, 17 February (www.kingsfund.org.uk/blog/2012/10/developing-culture-compassionate-care).

Courtenay, M., Nancarrow, S. and Dawson, D. (2013) 'Interprofessional teamwork in the trauma setting: a scoping review', *Human Resources for Health*, vol 11, no 1, p 57.

Curşeu, P.L. and Schreiber, S.G. (2010) 'Does conflict shatter trust or does trust obliterate conflict? Revisiting the relationship between team diversity, conflict and trust', *Group Dynamics: Theory Research and Practice*, vol 14, no 1, pp 66-79.

Dawson, J.F., West, M.A. and Yan, X. (2009) 'Positive and negative effects of team working in healthcare: "real" and "pseudo" teams and their impact on healthcare safety', Paper presented at the Annual National Clinical Assessment Service Conference, March.

de Bono, E. (1985) *Six thinking hats*, New York: Little, Brown & Company.

DH (Department of Health) (1998) *Partnership in action: New opportunities for joint working between health and social services*, London: DH.

DH (2000) *The NHS Plan: A plan for investment, a plan for reform*, London: The Stationery Office.

DH (2002) *Community mental health teams*, London: DH.

DH (2013) *Integrated care: Our shared commitment*, London: DH.

DH (2015a) *Learning not blaming: The government response to the Freedom to Speak Up consultation, the Public Administration Select Committee report 'Investigating clinical incidents in the NHS', and the Morecambe Bay Investigation*, London: DH.

DH (2015b) *Briefing note: Issues raised by the 2014 NHS Staff Survey in England* (www.nhsstaffsurveys.com/Page/1006/Latest-Results/2014-Results/).

Dickinson, H. (2014) *Performing governance: Partnerships, culture and New Labour*, Basingstoke: Palgrave Macmillan.

Dickinson, H. and Carey, G. (2016) *Managing and leading in inter-agency settings* (2nd edn), Better Partnership Working series, Bristol: Policy Press.

Dickinson, H. and O'Flynn, J. (2016) *Evaluating outcomes in health and social care* (2nd edn), Better Partnership Working series, Bristol: Policy Press.

Dixon-Woods, M., Baker, R., Charles, K., Dawson, J., Jerzembek, G., Martin, G. et al (2014) 'Culture and behaviour in the English National Health Service: overview of lessons from a large multimethod study', *British Medical Journal: Quality and Safety*, vol 23, pp 106-15.

Dunn, E., Mills, P., Neily, J., Crittenden, M., Carmack, A. and Baigan, J. (2007) 'Medical team training: applying crew resource management in the Veterans Administration', *The Joint Commission Journal on Quality and Patient Safety*, vol 33, pp 317-24.

Edmondson, A. (1996) 'Learning from mistakes is easier said than done: group and organisational influences on the detection and correction of human error', *Journal of Applied Behavioural Science*, vol 32, pp 5-28.

Edmondson, A. (2012) *Teaming: How organisations learn, innovate and compete in a knowledge economy*, Cambridge, MA: Harvard Business School Press.

Ellins, J. and Ham, C. (2009) *NHS mutual: Engaging staff and aligning incentives to achieve higher levels of performance*, London: Nuffield Trust.

Evans, S., Huxley, P., Baker, C., White, J., Madge, S., Onyett, S. and Gould, N. (2012) 'The social care component of multidisciplinary mental health teams: a review and national survey', *Journal of Health Services Research & Policy*, vol 17, suppl 2, pp 23-9.

Evetts, J. (1999) 'Professionalisation and professionalism: issues for interprofessional care', *Journal of Interprofessional Care*, vol 13, pp 119-28.

Fay, D., Borrill, C., Amir, Z., Haward, R. and West, M.A. (2006) 'Getting the most out of multidisciplinary teams: A multi-sample study of team innovation in health care', *Journal of Occupational and Organizational Psychology*, vol 79, no 4, pp 553-67.

Francis, R. (2010) *The Independent Inquiry into Care provided by Mid-Staffordshire NHS Foundation Trust, January 2005-March 2009*, London: HMSO.

Francis, R. (2013) *Report of the Mid Staffordshire NHS Foundation Trust Public Inquiry*, London: The Stationery Office.

Francis, R. (2015) *Freedom to speak up: An independent review into creating an open and honest reporting culture in the NHS*, London: HMSO.

Franklin, C.M., Bernhardt, J.M., Lopez, R.P., Long-Middleton, E.R. and Davis, S. (2015) 'Interprofessional teamwork and collaboration between community health workers and healthcare teams: An integrative review', *Health Services Research and Managerial Epidemiology*, vol 2, January-December.

Franx, G., Kroon, H., Grimshaw, J., Drake, R., Grol, R. and Wensing, M. (2008) 'Organizational change to transfer knowledge and improve quality and outcomes of care for patients with severe mental illness: a systematic overview of reviews', *Canadian Journal of Psychiatry*, vol 53, no 5, p 294.

Glasby, J. and Dickinson, H. (2014a) *Partnership working in health and social care: What is integrated care and how can we deliver it?* (2nd edn), Better Partnership Working series, Bristol: Policy Press.

Glasby, J. and Dickinson, H. (2014b) *A-Z of interagency working*, Basingstoke: Palgrave Macmillan.

Glendinning, C., Powell, M. and Rummery, K. (2002) *Partnerships, New Labour and the governance of welfare*, Bristol: Policy Press.

Gray, B., Sarnak, D. and Burgers, J. (2015) *Home care by self: Governing nursing teams: The Netherlands' Buurtzorg Model*, Washington, DC: The Commonwealth Fund, May.

Haig, K., Sutton, S. and Whittington, J. (2006) 'SBAR: a shared mental model to influence communication between clinicians', *Journal on Quality and Patient Safety*, vol 32, pp 167-75.

Haigh, R. (2004) 'The quintessence of an effective team: some development dynamics for staff groups', in P. Campling and R. Haigh (eds) *From toxic institutions to therapeutic environments*, London: Royal College of Psychiatrists, pp 119-30.

Hamman, W. (2004) 'The complexity of team training: what we have learned from aviation and its applications to medicine', *Quality and Safety in Health Care*, vol 13, pp 72-9.

Harvard Business Review (2011) *Building better teams*, Boston, MA: Harvard Business School Publishing Corporation.

Hawkins, P. (2014) *Leadership team coaching: Developing collective transformational leadership* (2nd edn), London: Kogan Page.

Hayes, P. (2011) *Leading and coaching teams to success: The secret life of teams*, Maidenhead: McGraw Hill.

Health and Social Care Information Centre (2014) *Data on written complaints in the NHS 2013-14*, Workforce and Facilities Team, Exeter: Health and Social Care Information Centre.

Hochschild, A.R. (1979) 'Emotion work, feeling rules, and social structure', *American Journal of Sociology*, vol 85, pp 551-75.

Home Office (2006) *Crime in England and Wales 2005/06*, London: Home Office.

Hudson, B. (2000) 'Inter-agency collaboration: a sceptical view', in A. Brechin, H. Brown and M. Eby (eds) *Critical practice in health and social care*, Milton Keynes: Open University Press, pp 253-74.

Huxley, P., Evans, S., Baker, C., White, J., Philpin, S., Onyett, S. and Gould, N. (2011) *Integration of social care staff within community mental health teams. Final report*, London: National Institute for Health Research (NIHR) Service Delivery and Organisation Programme.

Janis, I.L. (1972) *Victims of groupthink*, Boston, MA: Houghton Mifflin Company.

Jelphs, K. (2008) 'Reviewing the effectiveness of communication and associated aspects of team working in the Intensive Care Unit', Unpublished commissioned research.

Johnson, G., Scholes, K. and Whittington, R. (2008) *Exploring corporate strategy: Text and cases* (8th edn), New York: Pearson.

Johnston, S., Green, M., Thille, P., Savage, C., Roberts, L., Russell, G. and Hogg, W. (2011) 'Performance feedback: An exploratory study to examine the acceptability and impact for interdisciplinary primary care teams', *BMC Family Practice*, vol 12, no 1, p 14.

Jupp, B. (2000) *Working together: Creating a better environment for cross-sector partnerships*, London: Demos.

Katzenbach, J. and Smith, D. (1993) *The wisdom of teams: Creating the high-performance organization*, Boston, MA: Harvard Business School Press.

Ke, K.M., Blazeby, J.M., Strong, S., Carroll, F.E., Ness, A.R. and Hollingworth, W. (2013) 'Are multidisciplinary teams in secondary care cost-effective? A systematic review of the literature', *Cost Effectiveness and Resource Allocation*, vol 1, no 7, pp 1-13.

Kilmann, R.H. and Thomas, K.W. (1977) 'Developing a forced-choice measure of conflict-handling behavior: The "MODE" Instrument', *Education and Psychological Measurement*, vol 37, no 2, pp 309-25.

Kline, N. (2009) *More time to think: A way of being in the world*, London: Fisher King Publishing.

Laming, H. (2003) *The Victoria Climbié Inquiry: Report of an inquiry*, London: The Stationery Office.

Laming, W. (2009) *The protection of children in England: A progress report*, London: The Stationery Office.

Lasley, M. (2005) 'Difficult conversations: Authentic communication leads to greater understanding and teamwork', *Group Facilitation: A Research and Applications Journal*, vol 7, pp 13-20.

Leape, L. (1994) 'Error in medicine', *The Journal of the American Medical Association*, vol 272, pp 1851-7.

Lee, M. (2014) 'Leading virtual project teams: adapting leadership theories and communications techniques to 21st century organizations', *Project Management Journal*, vol, 45, no 4, p 3.

Lemieux-Charles, L. and McGuire, W.L. (2006) 'What do we know about health care team effectiveness? A review of the literature', *Medical Care Research and Review*, vol 63, no 3, pp 263-300.

Lencioni, P. (2002) *The five dysfunctions of a team*, San Francisco, CA: Jossey-Bass.

Lencioni, P. (2012) *The advantage: Why organizational health trumps everything else in business*, San Francisco, CA: Jossey-Bass.

Leonard, M., Graham, S. and Bonacum, D. (2004) 'The human factor: the critical importance of effective teamwork and communication in providing safe care', *Quality and Safety in Health Care*, vol 13, pp 85-90.

Leutz, W. (1999) 'Five laws for integrating medical and social services: lessons from the United States and the United Kingdom', *The Milbank Quarterly*, vol 77, no 1, pp 77-110.

Levy, P.F. (2001) 'The Nut Island effect: when good teams go wrong', *Harvard Business Review*, vol 9, pp 51-9.

Lingard, L. (2012) 'Productive complications: emergent ideas in team communication and patient safety', *Healthcare Quarterly,* vol 15, special issue, pp 18-23.

Lown, B. and Manning, C.F. (2010) 'The Schwartz Center Rounds: Evaluation of an interdisciplinary approach to enhancing patient-centred communication, teamwork and provider support', *Academic Medicine*, vol 85, no 6, pp 1073-81.

Lyubovnikova, J. and West, M. (2013) 'Why teamwork matters: Enabling health care team effectiveness for the delivery of high quality patient care', in E. Salas, S. Tannenbaum, D. Cohen and G. Latham (eds) *Developing and enhancing teamwork in organizations: Evidence-based best practices and guidelines* (vol 33), Oxford: John Wiley & Sons, pp 331-72.

Maben, J., Peccei, R., Adams, M., Robert, G., Richardson, A., Murrells, T. and Morrow, E. (2012) *Exploring the relationship between patients' experiences of care and the influence of staff motivation, affect and well-being*, London: National Institute for Health Research Service Delivery and Organisation Programme (www.nets.nihr.ac.uk/__data/assets/pdf_file/0007/85093/ES-08-1819-213.pdf).

McDonald, S. (2014) 'Organisational culture and the Bethanie Group: a case study on what works', *Psychology at Work* (http://pulseuk.org/wp-content/uploads/2014/10/Bethanie-Case-Study-FINAL.pdf)

Macleod, D. and Clarke, N. (2009) *Engaging for success: Enhancing performance through employee engagement*, London: Department for Business, Innovation and Skills.

McInnes, S., Peters, K., Bonney, A. and Halcomb, E. (2015) 'An integrative review of facilitators and barriers influencing collaboration and teamwork between general practitioners and nurses working in general practice', *Journal of Advanced Nursing*, vol 71, no 9, pp 1973-85.

McIntyre, R.M. and Salas, E. (1995) 'Measuring and managing for team performance: lessons from complex environments', in R.A. Guzzo and E. Salas (eds) *Team effectiveness and decision making in organizations*, San Francisco, CA: Jossey-Bass, pp 143-203.

Macy, B. and Izumi, H. (1993) 'Organizational change, design and work innovation: a meta-analysis of 131 North American field studies – 1961-1991', in W. Passmore and R. Woodman (eds) *Research in organizational change and design*, vol 7, Greenwich, CT: JAI Press, pp 235-313.

Mangan, C., Miller, R. and Ward, C. (2015) 'Knowing me, knowing you: inter-professional working between general practice and social care', *Journal of Integrated Care*, vol 23, no 2.

Maslin-Prothero, S.E. and Bennion, A.E. (2010) 'Integrated team working: a literature review', *International Journal of Integrated Care*, vol 10, April.

Martin, G.P. and Finn, R. (2011) 'Patients as team members: opportunities, challenges and paradoxes of including patients in multi-professional healthcare teams', *Sociology of Health & Illness*, vol 33, no 7, pp 1050-65.

Mehrabian, A. (1972) *Nonverbal communication*, Chicago, IL: Aldine-Atherton.

Miller, C., Freeman, M. and Ross, N. (2001) *Interprofessional practice in health and social care: Challenging the shared learning agenda*, London: Arnold.

Minkman, M.M.N., Ahaus, K.T.B. and Huijsman, R. (2009) 'A four phase development model for integrated care services in the Netherlands', *BMC Health Services Research*, vol 9, no 42 (http://bmchealthservres.biomedcentral.com/articles/10.1186/1472-6963-9-42).

Mitchell, R.J., Parker, V. and Giles, M. (2011) 'When do interprofessional teams succeed? Investigating the moderating roles of team and professional identity in interprofessional effectiveness', *Human Relations*, vol 64, no 10, pp 1321-43.

Mohrman, S.A., Cohen, S.G. and Mohrman, A.M. (1995) *Designing team-based organizations*, San Francisco, CA: Jossey-Bass.

Morrow, E., Robert, G. and Maben, J. (2014) 'Exploring the nature and impact of leadership on the local implementation of the Productive Ward Releasing Time to Care', *Journal of Health Organization and Management*, vol 28, no 2, pp 154-76.

Mueller, F., Proctor, S. and Buchanan, D. (2000) 'Team working in its context(s): antecedents, nature and dimensions', *Human Relations*, vol 3, pp 1387-424.

Nagpal, K., Arora, S., Vats, A., Wong, H., Sevdalis, N., Vincent, C. and Moorthy, K. (2012) 'Failures in communication and information transfer across the surgical pathway: interview study', *BMJ Quality & Safety*, vol 21, no 10, pp 843-9.

Natale, L. (2010) *Factsheet: Education in prisons*, London: Civitas.

NHS Future Forum (2012) *Integration: A report from the NHS Future Forum*, London: NHS Future Forum.

NHSME (National Health Service Management Executive) (1993) *Nursing in primary care – New world, new opportunities*, Leeds: NHSME.

O'Driscoll, W., Livingston, G., Lanceley, A., Nic a'Bháird, C., Xanthopoulou, P., Wallace, I. et al (2014) 'Patient experience of MDT care and decision-making', *Mental Health Review Journal*, vol 19, no 4, pp 265-78.

O'Leary, K.J., Sehgal, N.L., Terrell, G. and Williams, M.V. (2012) 'Interdisciplinary teamwork in hospitals: a review and practical recommendations for improvement', *Journal of Hospital Medicine*, vol 7, no 1, pp 48-54.

Øvretveit, J. (1995) 'Team decision making', *Journal of Interprofessional Care*, vol 9, pp 41-51.

Parker, R. and Bradley, L. (2000) 'Organisational culture in the public sector: evidence from six organisations', *The International Journal of Public Sector Management*, vol 13, pp 125-41.

Payne, M. (2000) *Teamwork in multiprofessional care*, Basingstoke: Macmillan.

Piper, P. and Ramos, M. (2006) 'A failure to communicate: Politics, scams and information flow during Hurricane Katrina', *The magazine for database professionals* (www.infotoday.com/searcher/jun06/Piper_Ramos.shtml).

Plsek, P. (1997) *Creativity, innovation and quality*, San Francisco, CA: ASQC Quality Press.

Porath, C. and Pearson, C. (2013) 'The price of incivility – lack of respect hurts morale – and the bottom line', *Harvard Business Review*, January-February, pp 115-21.

Prades, J., Remue, E., van Hoof, E. and Borras, J.M. (2015) 'Is it worth reorganising cancer services on the basis of multidisciplinary teams (MDTs)? A systematic review of the objectives and organisation of MDTs and their impact on patient outcomes', *Health Policy*, vol 119, no 4, pp 464-74.

Pritchard, K. and Eliot, J. (2012) *Help the helper: Building a culture of extreme teamwork*, New York: Penguin.

Reason, J. (2008) *The human contribution: Unsafe acts, accidents and heroic recoveries*, Farnham: Ashgate Publishing Company.

Reason, J. (2013) *A life in error – from little slips to big disasters*, Aldershot: Ashgate.

Reeves, S., Lewin, S., Espin, S. and Zwarenstein, M. (2011) *Interprofessional teamwork for health and social care* (vol 8), Oxford: John Wiley & Sons.

Reffo, G. and Wark, V. (2014) *Leadership PQ: How political intelligence sets successful leaders apart*, London: Kogan Page.

Rhodes, D. (2003) *Better informed? Inspection of the management and use of information in social care*, London: Department of Health.

Rice, A.H. (2000) 'Interdisciplinary collaboration in health care: Education, practice, and research', *National Academies of Practice Forum: Issues in Interdisciplinary Care*, January, London: Sage Publications.

Richardson, S. and Asthana, S. (2005) 'Policy and legal influences on inter-organisational information sharing in health and social care services', *Journal of Integrated Care*, vol 13, pp 3-10.

Richter, A.W., Dawson, J.F. and West, M.A. (2011) 'The effectiveness of teams in organizations: A meta-analysis', *The International Journal of Human Resource Management*, vol 22, no 13, pp 2749-69.

Robertson, I. and Cooper, C. (2011) *Well being: Productivity and happiness at work*, London: Palgrave Macmillan.

Rummery, K. and Glendinning, C. (2000) *Primary care and social services: Developing new partnerships for older people*, Abingdon: Radcliffe Medical Press.

Sakran, J.V., Finneman, B., Maxwell, C., Sonnad, S.S., Sarani, B., Pascual, J. et al (2012) 'Trauma leadership: does perception drive reality?', *Journal of Surgical Education*, vol 69, no 2, pp 236-40.

Salas, E., Burke, S.C. and Cannon-Bowers, J. (2000) 'Teamwork: emerging principles', *International Journal of Management Reviews*, vol 2, pp 339-56.

Sawbridge, Y. and Hewison, A. (2013) 'Thinking about the emotional labour of nursing: supporting nurses to care', *Journal of Health Organization and Management*, vol 27, no 1, pp 127-33.

Scandura, T.A. and Sharif, M.M. (2013) 'Team leadership: The Chilean mine case', in C.M. Giannantonio and A.E. Hurley-Hanson (eds) *Extreme leadership: Leaders, teams and situations outside the norm*, Northampton, MA: Edward Edgar Publishing, pp 131-40.

Schein, E. (2004) *Organizational culture and leadership*, San Francisco, CA: Jossey-Bass.

Schippers, M., West, M. and Dawson, J. (2015) 'Team reflexivity and innovation: The moderating role of team context', *Journal of Management*, vol 41, no 3, pp 769-88.

Seddon, J. (2004) 'It's the way we work ... not the people', *Personnel Today*, 16 March.

Sheehan, D., Robertson, L. and Ormond, T. (2007) 'Comparison of language used and patterns of communication in interprofessional and multidisciplinary teams', *Journal of Interprofessional Practice*, vol 21, pp 17-30.

Stanton, N. (2003) *Mastering communication*, Basingstoke: Palgrave Macmillan.

Sullivan, H. and Skelcher, C. (2002) *Working across boundaries: Collaboration in public services*, Basingstoke: Palgrave.

Sutcliffe, K., Lewton, E. and Rosenthal, M. (2004) 'Communication failures: an insidious contributor to medical mishaps', *Academy of Medicine*, February, vol 79, no 2, pp 186-94.

Sundstrom, E. (1999) *Supporting work team effectiveness: Best management practices for fostering high performance*, San Francisco, CA: Jossey-Bass.

Thomas, K.W. (2002) *Introduction to conflict management: Improving performance using the TKI*, Palo Alto, CA: Consulting Psychologists Press.

United States House of Representatives (2006) *A failure of initiative: Final report of the select bipartisan committee to investigate the preparation for and response to Hurricane Katrina*, Washington, DC: US Government Printing Office.

Weller, J., Frengley, R., Torrie, J., Shulruf, B., Jolly, B., Hopley, L. et al (2011) 'Evaluation of an instrument to measure teamwork in multidisciplinary critical care teams', *BMJ Quality & Safety*, vol 20, no 3, pp 216-22.

Welsh Assembly Government (2011) *Sustainable social services for Wales: A framework for action*, Cardiff: Welsh Assembly Government.

West, M.A. and Lyubovnikova, J. (2013) 'Illusions of team working in health care', *Journal of Health Organization and Management*, vol 27, no 1, pp 134-42.

West, M.A. and Markiewicz, L. (2006) *The effective partnership working inventory*, Working Paper, Birmingham: Aston Business School.

West, M.A., Borrill, C. and Unsworth, K. (1998) 'Team effectiveness in organizations', in C.L. Cooper and I.T. Robinson (eds) *International review of industrial and organizational psychology*, vol 13, Chichester: Wiley.

West, M.A., Dawson, J., Admasachew, L. and Topakas, A. (2013) *NHS staff management and health service quality* (www.gov.uk/government/uploads/system/uploads/attachment_data/file/215455/dh_129656.pdf).

West, M.A., Borrill, C., Dawson, J., Scully, J., Carter, M., Anelay, S. et al (2002) 'The link between the management of employees and patient mortality in acute hospitals', *International Journal of Human Resource Management*, vol 13, no 8, pp 1299-310.

West, M.A., Alimo-Metcalfe, B., Dawson, J., El Ansari, W., Glasby, J., Hardy, G. et al (2012) *Effectiveness of multi-professional team working (MPTW) in mental health care, Final report*, London: National Institute for Health Research (NIHR) Service Delivery and Organisation Programme.

Wholey, D.R., Disch, J., White, K.M., Powell, A., Rector, T.S., Sahay, A. and Heidenreich, P.A. (2014) 'Differential effects of professional leaders on health care teams in chronic disease management groups', *Health Care Management Review*, vol 39, no 3, pp 186-97.

Xyrichis, A. and Lowton, K. (2008) 'What fosters or prevents interprofessional teamworking in primary and community care? A literature review', *International Journal of Nursing Studies*, vol 45, no 1, pp 140-53.

Zwarenstein, M. and Reeves, S. (2000) 'What's so great about collaboration? We need more evidence and less rhetoric', *British Medical Journal*, vol 7241, pp 1022-3.

Index